Made Easy®
(Second MBBS Examination)

MBBS
Made Easy®
(Second MBBS Examination)

Second Edition

Manoj Vimal
MBBS (MD)
Maulana Azad Medical College
Associated Lok Nayak and GB Pant Hospitals and
Guru Nanak Eye Center
New Delhi, India
and
Lady Hardinge Medical College and
Associated Hospitals
New Delhi, India

JAYPEE BROTHERS MEDICAL PUBLISHERS (P) LTD
**New Delhi • Ahmedabad • Bengaluru • Chennai • Hyderabad
Kochi • Kolkata • Lucknow • Mumbai • Nagpur • St Louis (USA)**

Published by

Jitendar P Vij
Jaypee Brothers Medical Publishers (P) Ltd

Corporate Office
4838/24 Ansari Road, Daryaganj, **New Delhi** 110 002, India, Phone: +91-11-43574357

Registered Office
B-3 EMCA House, 23/23B Ansari Road, Daryaganj, **New Delhi** 110 002, India
Phones: +91-11-23272143, +91-11-23272703, +91-11-23282021
+91-11-23245672, Rel: +91-11-32558559, Fax: +91-11-23276490, +91-11-23245683
e-mail: jaypee@jaypeebrothers.com, Website: www.jaypeebrothers.com

Branches

❑ 2/B, Akruti Society, Jodhpur Gam Road Satellite
    Ahmedabad 380 015, Phones: +91-79-26926233, Rel: +91-79-32988717
    Fax: +91-79-26927094, e-mail: ahmedabad@jaypeebrothers.com
❑ 202 Batavia Chambers, 8 Kumara Krupa Road, Kumara Park East
    Bengaluru 560 001, Phones: +91-80-22285971, +91-80-22382956,
    +91-080-22372664, Rel: +91-80-32714073, Fax: +91-80-22281761
    e-mail: bangalore@jaypeebrothers.com
❑ 282 IIIrd Floor, Khaleel Shirazi Estate, Fountain Plaza, Pantheon Road
    Chennai 600 008, Phones: +91-44-28193265, +91-44-28194897
    Rel: +91-44-32972089, Fax: +91-44-28193231
    e-mail:chennai@jaypeebrothers.com
❑ 4-2-1067/1-3, 1st Floor, Balaji Building, Ramkote, Cross Road
    Hyderabad 500 095, Phones: +91-40-66610020, +91-40-24758498
    Rel: +91-40-32940929, Fax:+91-40-24758499
    e-mail: hyderabad@jaypeebrothers.com
❑ No. 41/3098, B & B1, Kuruvi Building, St. Vincent Road
    Kochi 682 018 Kerala, Phones: +91-484-4036109, +91-484-2395739
    +91-484-2395740, e-mail: kochi@jaypeebrothers.com
❑ 1-A Indian Mirror Street, Wellington Square
    Kolkata 700 013   Phones: +91-33-22651926, +91-33-22276404
    +91-33-22276415, Rel: +91-33-32901926, Fax: +91-33-22656075
    e-mail: kolkata@jaypeebrothers.com
❑ Lekhraj Market III, B-2, Sector-4, Faizabad Road, Indira Nagar
    Lucknow 226 016 Phones: +91-522-3040553, +91-522-3040554
    e-mail: lucknow@jaypeebrothers.com
❑ 106 Amit Industrial Estate, 61 Dr SS Rao Road, Near MGM Hospital, Parel
    Mumbai 400 012, Phones: +91-22-24124863, +91-22-24104532
    Rel: +91-22-32926896, Fax: +91-22-24160828
    e-mail: mumbai@jaypeebrothers.com
❑ "KAMALPUSHPA" 38, Reshimbag, Opp. Mohota Science College, Umred Road
    Nagpur 440 009, Phone: Rel: +91-712-3245220, Fax: +91-712-2704275
    e-mail: nagpur@jaypeebrothers.com

USA Office
1745, Pheasant Run Drive, Maryland Heights (Missouri), MO 63043, USA, Ph: 001-636-6279734
e-mail: jaypee@jaypeebrothers.com, anjulav@jaypeebrothers.com

MBBS Made Easy® (Second MBBS Examination)

© 2009, Manoj Vimal

This book has been published in good faith that the material provided by author is original. Every effort is made to ensure accuracy of material, but the publisher, printer and author will not be held responsible for any inadvertent error(s). In case of any dispute, all legal matters to be settled under Delhi jurisdiction only.

First Edition: 2002

Second Edition: **2009**

ISBN 978-81-8448-623-0

Typeset at   JPBMP typesetting unit
Printed at   Replika Press Pvt. Ltd.

To
My father
Shri BS Vimal

Foreword

Prof. A.S. Bais
M.S., F.I.M.S.A.
(Hon. Surgeon to President of India)
Principal and Medical Superintendent
प्रो० ए० एस० बैस
एम. एस., एफ. आई.एम.एस.ऐ.
(भारत के राष्ट्रपति के मानद सर्जन)
प्रधानाचार्य एवं चिकित्सा अधीक्षक

Government of India
Lady Hardinge Medical College & Associated Hospitals,
New Delhi-110001 (India)
भारत सरकार
लेडी हार्डिंग मेडिकल कालेज एवं सह अस्पताल
नई दिल्ली-110001 (भारत)
Phone : 3343984 Fax : 91-11-3340566
Grams : HARDONIAN

I have gone through the contents of the second edition of this book entitled **"MBBS Made Easy"** written by Dr Manoj Vimal of Maulana Azad Medical College, New Delhi.

It covers a wide range of subjects which gives a good understanding of the type of questions being asked in the examination and how to prepare for it. The effort is laudable as it helps considerably a student to overcome his anxiety and prepare for excellent result in the examination.

I wish Dr Manoj Vimal all success in his endeavour.

AS Bais

Foreword

Prof. A.S. Bais

I have gone through the contents of the second edition of this book entitled "MBBS Made Easy" written by Dr Manoj Vimal of Maulana Azad Medical College, New Delhi.

It covers a wide range of subjects, which gives a good understanding of the type of questions being asked in the examination and how to prepare for it. The effort is laudable as it helps considerably a student to overcome his anxiety and prepare for excellent result in the examination.

I wish Dr Manoj Vimal all success in his endeavour.

AS Bais

Foreword

Many medical students, after studying hard throughout the year, have difficulty in identifying and focusing on important topics while preparing for the university examination. They are not able to figure out what to anticipate during the examination and be prepared for it.

Dr Manoj Vimal, from his own experience while going through various examinations, and from that of others around him, has compiled a systematic list of important topics (along with brief solutions for some of them) on which the examination going candidate could concentrate. He has also indicated the part of the examination process (theory, viva, practical, etc.) and the type of format (short notes, long questions, explain why, drug of choice, etc.) in which that particular topic is likely to appear. The author has supplemented this with a framework of the pattern of examination with allocation of marks in different subjects; some university examination question papers as examples and an assortment of appendices containing information that is otherwise scattered. The whole purpose of the author is to familiarise the MBBS student with the examination system and help him in sailing through it.

Encouraged by the response that he got with the first edition, Dr Vimal has revised the booklet and made it more useful as well as user friendly. My blessings are with him.

Dr KD Tripathi

Preface

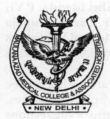

Manoj Vimal
MBBS MD (Std.)
Maulana Azad Medical College
Associated Lok Nayak and GB Pant Hospitals and
Guru Nanak Eye Center, New Delhi-110 002
Lady Hardinge Medical College and
Associated Hospitals, New Delhi-110 001
Resi: B-8/134, Sector-3, Rohini,
New Delhi-110 085, Ph: 09873388208
e-mail: manojvimal007@gmail.com
manojvimal007@yahoo.co.in

The aim of this book is to help the students appearing for second MBBS examination.

Special Features of the book are:
1. **Lucid language** and **up-to-date point coverage** of each and every subject.
2. This book will help the students to limit their reading and **"high yield"** in examination.
3. Covers both **new and old patterns** of examination followed throughout India.
4. This book will make the examination process **as simple as possible.**
5. This book provides all the information regarding second MBBS examination in a **systematic manner.**

This book is just an effort to help you during your examination. It will help you at **every step** throughout the whole process of examination. Special attractions like **drug of choice, laboratory diagnosis of some important infections, drugs in lactation, medicolegal aspect of forensic medicine, question papers for practice** and many more have also been covered in this book.

No effort of this kind is possible without generous cooperation and help of my colleagues, friends and teachers. My sincere thanks are due to all of them.

I wish to express gratitude to **my family, Dr AK Jain** (Professor of Physiology, MAMC) and **Dr Sushil Vimal** (Research Officer, Family Welfare Department, MAMC) for their sincere cooperation and encouragement.

I acknowledge with thanks my close friends **Shri Jitendar P Vij (Chairman and Managing Director) and Mr Tarun Duneja (Director-Publishing)** of M/s Jaypee Brothers Medical Publishers (P) Ltd, New Delhi for the assured cooperation and skills commendably used in preparing this book.

In spite of the best efforts, ventures of this kind are not likely to be free from human errors, inaccuracies and typographical mistakes. Therefore, I welcome a **feedback** from you in the form of **suggestions** for the further improvement of future editions of the book. Endeavour of this kind shall be **highly appreciated** and duly acknowledged. I hope this book will help you for preparing for your examinations.

Wishing you all the best for now and ever.

January, 2009   **Manoj Vimal**

Contents

PATHOLOGY

FORENSIC MEDICINE

APPENDICES

APPENDICES

PHARMACOLOGY

1. PATTERN OF EXAMINATION

PHARMACOLOGY	Marks
☞ Theory Paper I	40
☞ Theory Paper II	40
☞ Internal Assessment (Theory)	15
☞ Internal Assessment (Prac.)	15
☞ Prescription Writing	10
☞ Pharmacy Practical	5
☞ Clinical Case	5
☞ Experimental Pharmacology	10
☞ Theory Viva	10
Total	150

Note:

Paper I = * General Pharmacology
         * Autonomic Nervous System
         * Somatic Nervous System
         * Autacoids
         * Respiratory System
         * CNS and CVS
         * Kidney

Paper II = * Autacoids
         * Hormones
         * Blood and GIT
         * Antimicrobial Drugs
         * Anticancer Drugs

2. QUESTIONS FOR THEORY PAPER

A. GENERAL PHARMACOLOGY

SN: Half life of a drug (2005)

SN: Active transport

SN: Effect of food on absorption of drug

SN: Luminal effect

SN: Prodrug (1993)

SN: Why particle size of drug in a solid form is important in case of certain drugs like aspirin

SN: Clinical significance of volume distribution.

EW: Basic drugs are absorbed only when they reach intestine (2005)

SN: Types of adverse drug reactions (2004)

EW: Acidic drugs are poorly absorbed in alkaline medium

EW: Lipid soluble drugs are largely secreted unchanged

EW: Newborns are more susceptible to many drugs

SN: Factors affecting drug metabolism

SN: Clinical pharmacology

LQ: Routes of drug administration

LQ: Systemic routes of drug administration

SN: Pharmacogenomics (2004)

DW: Parenteral vs oral therapy

EW: Oral dose of some drugs are several fold higher than their parenteral done

EW: Action is faster via nasal route

SN: Fate of drug in body. Illustrate with example

SN: Microsomal enzyme induction

SN: First pass metabolism

SN: Discuss how drugs act through receptor

EW: A potent agonist antagonizes the action of full agonist

DW: Drug potency and efficiency

SN: Advantages and disadvantages of fixed done ratio combination

SN: Bioequivalence (2004)

SN: Factors modifying drug action

SN: Placebo

DW: Tolerance and resistance of drug

SN: Side effects

SN: Drug allergy
SN: Drug dependence
EW: Fixed dose combinations of drugs are often considered to be of disadvantage (2005)
SN: Tubular secretion of drugs
SN: Drug tolerance (2005)
SN: Clearance
SN: Plateau principle
SN: Principles of drug action
SN: Name drug which act by inhibiting enzymes
SN: Teratogenicity
SN: Essential medicines (2005)
SN: First dosage phenomenon (1991)
SN: Inverse agonist (1998)
EW: Half life of a drug varies for drugs undergoing zero order kinetics (2006)
SN: Polypharmacy (2006)
SN: Drug tolerance (2006)
SN: Pharmacovigilance (2006)
SN: Fixed dose drug combinations (2007)
SN: Drugs modulating cytochrome P_{450} enzymes (2007)
SN: Drug-dependence (2007)
SN: Therapeutic window (2008)
SN: Bioavailability (2008).

B. AUTONOMIC NERVOUS SYSTEM

LQ: Enumerate anticholinergic agents. Discuss their adverse effects and give their therapeutic based uses (2003)

EW: Pralidoxime is used in organophosphate poisoning and not in carbamate poisoning (2004)

SN: Uses and adverse effects of neostigmine

SN: Myasthenia gravis (2000)

SN: Treatment of organophosphorus poisoning

SN: Classification of anticholinergic drugs

SN: Uses of anticholinergic drugs

SN: Pralidoxime in organophosphorus poisoning (2005)

SN: Motion sickness

DW: Atropine and dopamine

DW: Adrenaline and ephedrine

EW: Large doses of acetylcholine causes increase in BP in atropinised animals

EW: Fenfluramine is used as anorectic over amphetamines

SN: Dopamine cardiogenic shock

EW: BAL is used in arsenic poisoning (2004)

SN: Anorectic agents

SN: Uses of α-blockers

SN: Effects of α blockers

EW: It is desirable to give phenoxybenzamine for 1-2 weeks preoperatively and continue it during surgery

SN: Propranolol

SN: Name cardioselective β blockers. How do these differ from nonselective in clinical terms

SN: Adverse effects of β blockers

SN: Uses of β blockers

EW: Acetylcholine is not used therapeutically

SN: Side effects of acetylcholine

EW: Pilocarpine is effective in acute congestive and simple glaucoma

SN: Pilocarpine

EW: Neostigmine but not physostigmine is used in myasthenia gravis

SN: Anticholinesterase

SN: Cholinergic drugs in Alzheimer's disease (2004)

EW: Atropine methonitrate is preferred to atropine sulphate as spasmolytic

SN: Mydriatics

TS: Adrenaline in anaphylactic shock

SN: Cardiac and metabolic effects of synthetic amines

SN: Classify adrenergic drugs

SN: Dopamine

LQ: Classify adrenergic blocking agents. Discuss indications and contraindications with reasoning of β adrenergic blocking agent

EW: Propranolol but not atenolol is used for treatment of tremors (2003)

SN: Beta adrenergic blockers in angina pectoris (2004)

DT: Benign hyperplasia of prostate (2005)

EW: Atropine is preferred for refraction testing in children (2006)

TS: Tamsulosin in benign prostatic hypertrophy (2006)

Que: Discuss rationale for the use of finasteride in benign prostatic hyperstrophy (2006)

EW: First dose of prazosin should preferably be administered at bed time (2007)

Que: Give rationale for the therapeutic use of oximes in organophosphorus poisoning (2007)

Que: Give rationale for the use of BAL in arsenic poisoning (2007)

Que: Give rationale for the use of sildenafil in erectile dysfunction (2007)

Que: Give rationale for the use of finasteride in prostatic disease (2007)

Que: Give the rationale for the therapeutic use of sildenafil in erectile dysfunction (2008).

C. SOMATIC NERVOUS SYSTEM

SN: Peripherally acting muscle relaxants (classification)

TS: Lignocaine

SN: Bupivacaine

EW: oxethiazine is a good anaesthesia for gastric mucosa while other local anaesthetise are not

DW Competitive and depolarizing block

SN: Beclofen

SN: Uses of centrally acting muscles relaxants

SN: Classify local anaesthetics

EW: d-tubocuranine produces significant fall in BP

EW: Neuromuscular blockers not absorbed orally

EW: Thiopentone sodium and succinylcholines solutions should not be mixed in the same syringe

TS: Dentrolene

LQ: Centrally acting muscle relaxants

TS: Diazepam

EW: Addition of vasoconstrictor to local anaesthetic

DW: Procaine and lignocaine

SN: Uses of local anaesthesia

SN: Epidural anaesthesia

SN: Spinal anaesthesia (1998)

EW: Pralidoxime is ineffective as antidote to carbamate poisoning (2006)

Que: Give rationale for the therapeutic use of tizanidine in spastic disorders (2007)

EW: Dose of skeletal muscle relaxant should be lowered in patients receiving high doses of gentamicin (2007).

D. AUTACOIDS

TS: Ondansetron as an antiemetic (2002)
SN: 5-HT antagonist
LQ: Angiotensin converting enzyme inhibitors
SN: Enalapril
DW: H1, H2 and H3 receptors
SN: Name the actions of histamine not antagonised by antihistamine
SN: H1 antagonist and their use
SN: Cetrizine
SN: Second generation antihistaminics (2001)
SN: Cinnarizine
EW: Enalapril is preferred over captopril
SN: Uses of ACE inhibitors
TS: Prostaglandin in obstetrics
EW: Aspirin is used in children having patent ductus arteriosus
EW: Prostaglandins are not considered as neurotransmitters
SN: Leukotrienes
TS: Prostaglandins for inducing therapeutic action
EW: Finasteride is used in benign hypertrophy of prostate (2001)
SN: Ondansetron in chemotherapy induced vomiting (2004)
Que: Discuss the drug treatment of migraine (2006)
Que: 5 HT$_3$ antagonists in vomiting (2006)
Que: Give rationale for the therapeutic use of sumatriptan in migraine (2007).

E. RESPIRATORY SYSTEM

SN: Ipratropium bromide in chronic obstructive pulmonary disease (2005)

TS: Salbutamol (1991)

SN: Terbutaline

EW: Aminophylline is given by slow IV injection

SN: Sodium chromoglycate

SN: KI (potassium iodide)

SN: Mucolytics

SN: Name the drug of choice in prophylaxis of chronic bronchial asthma

TS: Inhalational steroids in bronchial asthma

SN: Antitussives

SN: Treatment of cough

SN: Give a plan of action for treatment of bronchial asthma (1998)

EW: Antihistamine not used for treatment of bronchial asthma

EW: Salbutamol is preferred over isoprenaline for treatment of acute bronchial asthma

EW: Inhalation, administration of β2 agonist is preferred to oral administration is asthma

EW: Aminophylline is not used in treatment of angina pectoris

TS: Corticosteroids in bronchial asthma

SN: Treatment of status asthmatics (2001)

TS: Ephedrine in cough syrup (2006)

Que: Discuss the drug treatment of status asthmaticus (2007)

TS: Leukotriene antagonists in bronchial asthma (2007)

TS: Sodium chromoglycate in bronchial asthma (2008).

F. HORMONES

LQ: Classify oral contraceptives. Discuss the mechanism of action, adverse effects and contraindication of oral contraceptives (2005)

SN: Mechanism of action of insulin

EW: Regular insulin is not combined with lente insulin (2005)

EW: Mifepristone is used for therapeutic abortion (2005)

EW: Insulin induced hypoglycemia may be affected by concurrent administration of salisalates

SN: Classify drugs used in diabetes mellitus with mechanism of action and side effects

SN: Management of diabetic ketoacidosis

SN: Insulin resistance

EW: Oral hypoglycemic agents are ineffective in juvenile diabetes mellitus

TS: Human insulin

SN: Oxytocin (2005)

SN: Mechanism of action of steroidal hormones

SN: Bromocriptine

LQ: Thyroid hormones and their uses

SN: Management of thyrotoxicosis

SN: Classify drugs used in thyroid disorders. Discuss status of iodine

SN: Myxoedema coma

SN: Antithyroid drugs

LQ: Carbimazole

EW: Iodides are not used for long-term treatment of hyper-thyroidism

EW: Prophylthiouracil is preferred over methimazole in treatment of thyroid storm

EW: Lugol's iodine has a limited use as an antithyroid drug
Describe the rationale the drug treatment of hyperthyroidism (2001)

SN: Radioactive iodine

SN: Potassium iodide in thyrotoxicosis (2002)

SN: Raloxifene in osteoporosis (2005)

SN: Diabetic ketoacidosis (2002)

SN: More purified insulin preparations

LQ: Oral hypoglycemia drugs

TS: Sulfonylureas

Que: Describe the mechanism of action of sulfonylureas (2001)

SN:　Treatment of sulfonylurea induced hypoglycemia

SN:　Pharmacological basis of use of tolbutamide in maturity onset DM (NIDDM)

EW:　Biguanides not used in underweight patient with NIDDM

SN:　Mechanism of action of biguanides

SN:　Status of oral hypoglycemics in DM

Que:　Describe the rationale the drug treatment of postmenopausal syndrome and osteoporosis (2001)

TS:　Biguanids in diabetes mellitus (2002)

SN:　Antiandrogens (2002)

LQ:　Corticosteroids (actions and uses)

SN:　Clomiphene in treatment of infertility (2005)

SN:　Anti-inflammatory effects of corticosteroids

EW:　Glucocorticoids, mechanism of action

DW　Synthetic and natural adrenal corticosteroids

DW　Hydrocortisone and dexamethasone

SN:　Prednisolone

SN:　Replacement therapy

EW:　Corticosteroids are administered in tubercular meningitis

TS:　Corticosteroids in autoimmune diseases

TS:　Corticosteroids in eye diseases

SN:　Explain effect of sudden withdrawal of steroids in bronchial asthma and mechanism involved

EW:　Corticosteroids cause less suppression of pituitary axis if given at 7.00 in morning

SN:　Side effects of androgens

SN:　Rosiglitazone in diabetes mellitus (2005)

EW:　Use of anabolic steroid is on decline

SN:　Uses of anabolic steroids

TS:　Anabolic steroids

SN:　Antiandrogens

EW:　Use of short-term high dose estrogen is not recommended to test pregnancy

SN:　Delayed puberty in girls

TS:　Antiestrogens, e.g. clomiphene citrate

TS:　Tamoxifen citrate

EW:　Progestins added to estrogens in oral contraceptive pills whereas estrogen alone can produce contraception

SN:　Long-term antifertility agents.

EW:　Progesterone is added with oestrogen for hormone replacement therapy (2002)

SN:　Female contraception

SN: Oral contraceptives

SN: Postcoital pill

LQ: Classify adrenocorticosteroids. Discuss the pharmacological actions, side effects, contraindications and therapeutic uses of glucocorticoids (2004)

EW: Estrogen in high doses is effective as postcoital contraception

EW: Ethinyloestradiol and not estradiol is used in oral contraception preparation

SN: Mechanism of injectable contraceptives

SN: Side effects of hormonal contraceptives

SN: Male contraceptives

SN: Postcoital (emergency) contraception (2001)

SN: Oxytocin

SN: Uterine stimulants

SN: Tocolytics

SN: Calcium antagonists and calcium channel blockers

EW: Vitamin D should be considered as hormone

Que: Describe the rationale the drug treatment of hyperthyroidism (2001)

DT: Thyrotoxicosis crisis (2005)

EW: Bisphosphonates are often prescribed to postmenopausal women (2006)

EW: Lispro insulin is used in infusion pump devices (2006)

Que: Discuss rationale for the use of progesterone with oestrogen in hormone replacement therapy (2006)

Que: Discuss rationale for the use of mifiprestone for termination of early pregnancy (2006)

SN: Selective oestrogen receptor modulators (2006)

Que: Classify drugs used in diabetes mellitus. Describe the pharmacology of oral hypoglycemic drugs (2007)

TS: Bisphosphonates in osteoporosis (2007)

TS: Tamoxifen in breast cancer (2007)

SN: Emergency contraceptives (2007)

Que: Explain why oxytocin and not ergometrine is used for augmenting the labour (2008)

Que: Give the rationale for the use of propranolol in thyrotoxicosis (2008)

Que: Give the rationale for the use of alendronate in osteoporosis (2008)

TS: Rosiglitazone in diabetes mellitus (2008)

SN: Emergency contraception (2008)

G. CENTRAL NERVOUS SYSTEM

SN: Objectives of general anaesthesia

SN: Factors affecting the partial pressure of anaesthetic attained in brain

SN: Classify intravenous anaesthetics. Outline their role in anaesthetic practice

EW: N_2O is not considered as complete anaesthetic in abdominal operations

ENU   General anaesthetics

SN: N_2O

SN: Ether

EW: Enflurane is preferred over methoxyflurane

SN: Halothane

EW: Plasma concentration of phenytoin rises disproportionably at higher doses (2005)

SN: Recovery with thiopentone is rapid

EW: Neurolept analgesic should not be used in person with parkinsonism

EW: Dose of d-Tc is reduced to half in treatment with ether

SN: Complications of general anaesthesia

SN: Preanaesthetic medication

SN: Acute alcohol intoxication

TS: Disulfiram

SN: Disulfiram

SN: Treatment of methyl alcohol poisoning

LQ: Benzodiazepines

EW: Benzodiazepines are preferred over barbiturates as hypnotics (2003)

EW: Dose of phenobarbitone sodium is increased in treatment of neonatal jaundice

TS: Barbiturates

SN: Acute barbiturate poisoning

SN: Uses of diazepam

EW: Benzodiazepines are preferred over barbiturates as hypnotics

SN: Flumazenil

SN: Classify antiepileptic drugs

SN: Levodopa and carbidopa combination in parkinsonism (2005)

TS: Phenobarbitone as antiepileptic drug

SN: Phenytoin

SN: Carbamazepine
SN: Treatment of epilepsy
SN: Treatment of GTCS
SN: Treatment of status epilepticus
TS: Levodopa in parkinsonism
DT: Status epilepticus (2005)
SN: Advantages of carbidopa over levodopa
TS: Bromocriptine in epilepsy
SN: Treatment of drug induced parkinsonism
SN: Selegiline
EW: Combination of L-dopa and carbidopa is ineffective in drug-induced parkinsonism
SN: Classify antipsychotic drugs
SN: Mechanism of action of chlorpromazine
SN: Olanzapine in schizophrenia (2004)
EW: Chlorpromazine is not used as local anaesthetic instead of being more potent than procaine
SN: Enumerate drugs in order of preference which you would like to give in treatment of psychoses
SN: Haloperidol
LQ: Classify drugs used in mental illness. Give actions and adverse effects of chlorpromazine
SN: Pimozide
EW: Chlorpromazine is not used routinely for anxiety though it has antianxiety activity
EW: Chlorpromazine is not used in motion sickness
SN: Treatment of psychoses
SN: Classify antianxiety drugs. Discuss diazepam
SN: Buspirone
LQ: Antidepressants
EW: Tricyclic antidepressants are preferred over noradrenaline inhibitors for endogenous depression
EW: Use of physostigmine in treatment of overdose of tricyclic anti-depressants
TS: Fluoxetine in depression
SN: Treatment of endogenous depressions
SN: Lithium carbonate
SN: Opioid analgesics, uses and adverse effects
TS: Morphine as analgesic
EW: Morphine is contraindicated in head injury and bronchial asthma

SN: Acute morphine poisoning
SN: Pethidine
TS: Tramadol as analgesic
SN: Cardiac asthma
SN: Pentazocine
SN: Naloxone
LQ: Classify NSAIDs. Give uses and adverse effects
SN: Aspirin
EW: Aspirin causes gastric bleeding
SN: Phenylbutazone
SN: Indomethacin
SN: Ibuprofen
SN: Mephenamic acid
SN: Diclofenac sodium
SN: Ketorolac
SN: Treatment of acute paracetamol poisoning
TS: Gold in rheumatoid arthritis
SN: Treatment of rheumatoid arthritis
SN: Treatment of acute gout
SN: Chronic gout
SN: Allopurinol
EW: Allopurinol is preferred over probenecid for chronic gout
SN: Pyritinol
LQ: Classify the drugs used in treatment of psychosis. Discuss the mechanism of action, side effects with their management and therapeutic uses of haloperidol (2004)
Que: Give rationale for the use of diazepam in tetanus (2006)
Que: Give rationale for the use of sodium bicarbonate in salicylate poisoning (2006)
Que: Discuss the drug treatment of status epilepticus (2006)
EW: Ethanol is used in methanol poisoning (2007)
EW: Plasma concentration of phenytoin rises disproportionately at higher doses (2007)
Que: Classify antidepressant drugs. Write the mechanism of action, adverse effects and therapeutic uses of fluoxetine (2007)
Que: Discuss the drug treatment of paracetamol poisoning (2007)
EW: Thalidomide is used for lepra reaction (2007)
Que: Give rationale for the use of hydroxychloroquine in systemic lupus erythematosis (2007).

Que: Explain why diazepam though a drug of choice for status epilepticus is not recommended for maintenance therapy of epilepsy (2008)

Que: Explain why halothane is frequently combined with nitrous oxide for general anesthesia (2008)

LQ: Enumerate commonly used opioids. Write the mode of action, indications and contraindications for the use of morphine (2008)

Que: Give the rationale for the therapeutic use of combining levodopa with carbidopa in parkinsonism (2008)

Que: Discuss the drug treatment of generalized tonic clonic seizures (2008)

Que: Discuss the drug treatment of acute gout (2008)

TS: Clozapine in schizophrenia (2008)

SN: Midazolam (2008).

H. CARDIOVASCULAR SYSTEM

LQ: Classify antihypertensive drugs. Discuss the mechanism of action, side effects and therapeutic uses of enalapril (2005)

EW: Enalapril should not be give concurrently with triamterene (2003)

SN: Treatment of atrial fibrillation

LQ: Classify antiarrhythmic drugs give mechanism of action

EW: Paroxysmal tachycardia due to quinidine occurs only in patients of atrial fibrillation

TS: Lignocaine as antiarrhythmic drugs

LQ: Cardiac glycosides

SN: Digoxin induced cardiac toxicity

SN: Drug treatment of cardiogenic shock

SN: Drug treatment of congestive heart failure

TS: Vasodilatation in CHF

EW: Alteplase is used in the treatment of myocardial infarction (2002)

EW: Digitalis is used in atrial fibrillation

TS: Digitalis in CHF

SN: Amiodarone

TS: Verapamil in arrhythmia

EW: Verapamil is not given with propranolol

SN: Lignocaine in ventricular arrhythmias (2005)

EW: There is marked difference in action of verapamil and nifedipine whereas both are calcium channel blockers

SN: Treatment of angina pectoris

EW: Aminophylline is not used in treatment of angina pectoris

EW: Propranolol is not used in vasospastic angina

EW: Streptokinase is used in the treatment of myocardial infarction (2004)

SN: Classify antianginal drugs

TS: Glycerol trinitrate

EW: Nifedipine causes headache

TS: Calcium channel blockers as antianginal drugs

SN: Amlodipine

EW: Drug free period is advocated for transdermal nitroglycerine therapy in patients suffering from angina pectoris (2003)

TS: Dipyridamole

SN: Management of myocardial infarction

SN: Classify antihypertensive drugs

EW: Dopamine is used in the management of shock (2004)

TS: Calcium channel blockers in hypertension

TS: Thiazides in hypertension

SN: Indications and drawbacks of using furosemide in hypertension

SN: Use of hydralazine in HT

SN: Treatment of hypertension

SN: Hypertension in pregnancy

Que: Discuss the therapeutic status of thrombolytic agents in myocardial infarctions (2001)

SN: Cavedilol in hypertension (2004)

DT: Hypertensive emergencies (2004)

Que: Give rationale for the therapeutic use of adenosine in the treatment of paroxysmal atrial tachycardia (2007)

TS: ACE inhibitors in heart failure (2007)

EW: Digoxin is contraindicated in Wolf-Parkinson-White syndrome (2006)

Que: Enumerate drugs for the treatment of congestive heart failure Discuss the mechanism of action, therapeutic uses and adverse effects of enalapril (2006)

Que: Give rationale for the use of carvidelol in heart failure (2006)

Que: Give rationale for the use of adenosine in supraventricular tachycardia (2006)

Que: Explain why digoxin but not adrenaline is used in congestive heart failure (2008)

Que: Give the rationale for the therapeutic use of dopamine in cardiogenic shock (2008).

I. KIDNEY, BLOOD AND GIT

SN: Classify diuretics, also give uses

EW: Furosemide is used in the treatment of acute pulmonary edema (2004)

SN: Frusemide

SN: Complications of diuretic therapy

SN: Potassium sparing diuretics

EW: Thiazides are used in diabetes insipidus (2004)

SN: Drug treatment of microcytic hypochromic anaemia

EW: Furosemide is also known as a high ceiling diuretic (2005)

SN: Management of acute iron poisoning

EW: Both folate and Vitamin B_{12} deficiency produces several common manifestations

EW: Vitamin B_{12} is preferred over folic acid for treatment of pernicious anaemia

SN: Folic acid

EW: Vitamin B_{12} is administered parenterally in patients of pernicious anaemia (2002)

SN: *H. pylori* infection (2002)

EW: Use of folinic acid with methotrexate

SN: Vitamin K

SN: Warfarin (2002)

EW: Vitamin K_1 used to reverse overdose of oral anticoagulants

SN: Anticoagulants

EW: Oral anticoagulants take days to act while heparin takes minute

SN: Heparin

SN: Oral anticoagulants

SN: Treatment of bleeding due to oral anticoagulants

EW: Cefoperazone should be used cautiously in patients on anticoagulant therapy (2005)

EW: Oral anticoagulants should not be used in pregnancy

SN: Fibrinolytic therapy

SN: Streptokinase

EW: Streptokinase has little or no benefit if infused after 12 hours of onset of symptoms in MI

TS: Antifibrinolytics

TS: Aspirin as antithrombotic drugs

SN: Uses of antiplatelet drugs

SN: Clofibrate

SN: Gemfibrozil

EW: Clofibrate is used in hyperlipoproteinemia

TS: Lovastatin as hypolipidemic drug

SN: Statins in dyslipidemia (2005)

SN: Uses of plasma expanders

Que: Discuss the therapeutic status of Sulfasalazine in ulcerative colitis (2001)

SN: Classify drugs used for treatment of peptic ulcer

SN: Ranitidine

TS: Omeprazole in peptic ulcer

SN: Erythropoietin in chronic renal failure (2005)

EW: Loperamide should be avoided in treatment of infective diarrhoea (2004)

SN: Five important properties of an ideal antacid

EW: Magnesium trisilicate is used in treatment of peptic ulcer

EW: Aluminium hydroxide is used with $Mg(OH)_2$ in antacid gel

Que: Describe the rationale the drug treatment of *H.pylori* associated upper gastrointestinal disorders (2001)

TS: Carbenoxolone sodium

EW: Mesna is used with ifosfamide (2005)

SN: Cinnarizine

SN: Metoclopramide

TS: Domperidone

SN: Cisapride

SN: Stimulant purgatives

SN: Bisacodyl

SN: Purgative abuse

SN: Treatment of diarrhoea

SN: Oral rehydration therapy

EW: Use of glucose in ORS

SN: Diphenoxylate

Que: Describe the mechanism of action of purgatives (2001)

Que: Describe the rationale the drug treatment of *H.pylori* associated upper gastrointestinal disorders (2001)

Que: Describe the mechanism of action of purgatives (2001)

DT: Postoperative paralytic ileus (2005)

SN: Rofecoxib as anti-inflammatory (2005)

EW: Ketoconazole should not be used with cisapride (2006)

EW: Low molecular weight heparins are preferred over unfractionated heparin preparations (2006)

Que: Discuss rationale for the use of corticosteroids in ulcerative colitis (2006)

Que: Discuss the drug treatment of peptic ulcer (2006)

TS: Folic acid in anaemia (2006)

EW: Thiazide diuretics cause calcium retention while loop diuretics cause increase in calcium excretion (2007)

TS: Statins in dyslipidemia

EW: Heparin and Warfarin are started together in acute thromboembolic states (2007)

Que: Explain why acetazolamide is not r referred as a diuretic agent (2008)

Que: Give the rationale for the therapeutic use of mannitol in cerebral oedema (2008)

TS: Terlipress in bleeding oesophageal varices (2008)

Que: Explain why ondansetron is preferred over prochlor-perazine for the treatment of cancer chemotherapy induced emesis (2008)

Que: Discuss the drug treatment of peptic Ulcer with H. pylori infection (2008)

SN: Plasma expanders (2008).

J. ANTIMICROBIAL DRUGS

SN: Classify antimicrobial drugs

Que: Describe the factors which govern the selection of an antimicrobial drug for treatment of infections (2001)

SN: Drug resistance

EW: Penicillin is lethal to bacterial cell but *practicaly* non-toxic to mammalian cell (2002)

SN: Suprainfection

SN: Advantages and disadvantages of combined use of antimicrobials

Que: Describe the mechanism of action of aminoglycoside antibiotics (2001)

SN: Prophylactic use of antimicrobials

Que: Describe the mechanism of action of aminoglycoside antibiotics (2001)

SN: Adverse effects of sulfonamides

SN: Uses of cotrimoxazole

EW: Sulphadoxine is combined with pyrimethamine (2004)

SN: Trimethoprim

SN: Ciprofloxacin, uses and adverse effects

SN: Mechanism of action of penicillins

SN: Adverse effects of penicillin specially hypersensitivity

SN: Uses of penicillins

SN: Semisynthetic penicillin

SN: Ampicillin

SN: Amoxicillin

Que: Discuss the therapeutic status of metronidazole in anaerobic infections (2001)

SN: Beta lactamase inhibitors

SN: Sulbactam

LQ: Cephalosporins, classification, mechanism of the action, uses and adverse effects

SN: Third generation cephalosporins

LQ: Classify tetracyclines, mechanism of action, uses and adverse effects of tetracyclines also give precautions before prescribing tetracycline

SN: Chloramphenicol

LQ: Give properties, mech. of action, toxicities and uses of aminoglycoside antibiotics

SN: Streptomycin

SN: Amikacin

SN: Neomycin

SN: Erythromycin

SN: Roxithromycin

SN: Nitrofurantoin

SN: Treatment of urinary tract infections

SN: Fluoroquinolones in tuberculosis (2005)

SN: Classify antitubercular drugs

SN: Isoniazid

SN: Rifampicin

SN: Acyclovir in herpes infections (2005)

SN: Ethambutol

SN: Pyrazinamide

SN: Treatment of tuberculosis

SN: Short course chemotherapy

SN: Lamotrigine in epilepsy (2004)

TS: Corticosteroids in treatment of tuberculosis

TS: Fluoroquinolones in tuberculosis (2002)

SN: Clofazimine

TS: Rifampicin in leprosy

SN: Multibacillary leprosy (2002)

SN: Treatment of leprosy

SN: Multidrug therapy of leprosy

TS: Amphotericin B in fungal infections

SN: Azole anti-fungal agents (2001)

SN: Griseofulvin

DT: Multi-bacillary leprosy (2005)

SN: Clotrimazole

TS: Ketoconazole

SN: Fluconazole

SN: Acyclovir

SN: Zidovudine

SN: Interferon α

EW: Classify drugs used in the treatment of malaria. Discuss the pharmacology of chloroquine and mefloquin (2002)

SN: Classify antimalarial drugs

SN: Radical treatment of malaria

LQ: Chloroquine

TS: Mefloquine

TS: Quinine

SN: Pyrimethamine

SN: Primaquine

SN: Classify antiamoebic drugs

SN: Metronidazole

SN: Metronidazole in the management of pseudomembranous colitis (2002)

SN: Imipenem in combination with cilastatin (2002)

TS: Chloroquine as antiamoebic drug

SN: Diloxanide furoate

TS: Mebendazole

SN: Albendazole

TS: Pyrantel pamoate

SN: Ivermectin

SN: Niclosamide

SN: Praziquantel

EW: Cisapride should not be used in patients receiving erythromycin (2001)

EW: Use of mefloquin is restricted to areas where chloroquine resistance is prevalent (2001)

SN: Directly observed treatment strategy (DOTS) for tuberculosis (2005)

SN: Quinine in cerebral malaria (2005)

Que: Enumerate aminoglycoside antibiotics. Discuss their mechanism of action, anti-bacterial spectrum, therapeutics uses and side effects (2006)

TS: Fluoroquinolones in tuberculosis (2006)

SN: Irrational use of antimicrobial agents (2006)

SN: Macrolide antibiotics (2006)

EW: Anaerobic microorganisms are resistant to aminoglycoside antibiotics (2007)

Que: Discuss the drug treatment of MDR tuberculosis (2007)

TS: Cyclosporine in renal transplants (2007)

SN: Albendazole (2007)

Que: Explain why ketoconazole is useful in treatment of Cushing's syndrome (2008)

Que: Give the rationale for the use of diloxanide furoate and metronidazole in amoebiasis (2008)

Que: Discuss the drug treatment of chronic, recurrent urinary tract infection in females (2008)

LQ: What is HAART? Write the mode of action, adverse effects and clinically important drug interactions of nevirapine (2008)

TS: Ivermectin in filariasis (2008)

TS: Artemisinin in malaria (2008)

SN: Post antibiotic effect (2008)

K. ANTICANCER DRUGS

SN: Classify anticancer drugs
SN: General toxicity of cytotoxic drugs
SN: Ondansetron in chemotherapy induced vomiting (2004)
SN: Tamoxifen in the treatment of carcinoma breast (2002)
SN: Nucleoside reverse transcriptase inhibitors (2005)
SN: Cyclophosphamide
SN: Methotrexate
SN: Methotrexate in rheumatoid arthritis (2005)
SN: Vincristine
SN: Rubidomycin
SN: 5-FU (5-Fluorouracil)
SN: Tamoxifen in breast cancer (2004)
DT: Emesis due to cancer chemotherapy (2005)
Que: Discuss the drug treatment of HIV infection (2007)
SN: Paclitaxel (2007)
Que: Explain why dexrazoxane pretreatment is given with doxorubicin therapy (2008)
Que: Give the rationale for the use of filgrastim in cancer chemotherapy (2008).

L. MISCELLANEOUS DRUGS

SN: Vitamin A (2002)
EW: Deficiencies of folic acid and vitamin B_{12} have many common features (2001)
SN: Action of kaolin on GIT
SN: Astringents
DW: Irritants and counter irritants
SN: Mechanism of counter irritation pain relief
SN: Keratolytics
SN: Melanizing agents
SN: Sunscreens
SN: Treatment of acne vulgaris
SN: Topical steroids
DW   Antiseptics and disinfectants
SN: Role of antiseptics in hospitals
SN: Cetrimide
SN: Drug of choice for mercury poisoning
SN: Penicillamine
SN: Desferrioxamine
DW   Retinol and retinoic acid
SN: Vitamin E
DW   Calcitonin and vitamin D
SN: Hypervitaminosis A
SN: TAB vaccines
SN: Hepatitis B vaccine
SN: DPT vaccine
Que: Discuss the drug treatment of scabies (2006).

Note:
LQ: Long Questions
SN: Short Note
DW: Difference Between
EW: Explain Why
TS: Therapeutic Status
DT: Drug Treatment
Que: Question
ENU: Enumeration
Nm: Normal
Abn: Abnormal

3. TOPICS FOR PRESCRIPTION WRITING

1. Treatment of pulmonary tuberculosis
2. Treatment of bronchial asthma
3. Treatment of peptic ulcer
4. Treatment of scabies
5. Treatment of infective diarrhoea
6. Treatment of congestive heart failure
7. Treatment of non-productive cough
8. Treatment of hypertension
9. Treatment of malaria (Both presumptive and radical)
10. Treatment of migraine
11. Treatment of meningitis
12. Treatment of myocardial infarction
13. Treatment of pneumonia
14. Treatment of sinusitis
15. Treatment of UTI.

4. TOPICS FOR PHARMACY PRACTICAL

You are provided raw material and allowed to prepare the drug and you are supposed to know:

- Method of preparation
- Uses
- Leading questions

Drugs

1. Calamine lotion
2. Mendel's paint
3. ORS
4. Carminative mixture.

5. TOPICS FOR EXPERIMENTAL PRACTICAL

An experimental animal, e.g. frog, rabbit, cat's ileum to provided to you and you are asked to demonstrate the effects of various drugs on these animals or organs of the animals:

1. Frog's heart
2. Rectus abdominis of frog
3. Ileum of cat
4. Rabbit's eye.

6. TOPICS FOR THEORY VIVA

⇨ Various routes of drug administration
⇨ First pass metabolism
⇨ Plasma half life
⇨ Plateau principal
⇨ Drug potency and efficacy
⇨ Side effects of drug
⇨ Muscarinic and nicotinic receptors
⇨ Treatment of migraine
⇨ Cholinergic and anticholinergic drugs
⇨ Atropine
⇨ Adrenaline in anaphylactic shock
⇨ Centrally acting muscle relaxants
⇨ Uses and limitations of local anaesthetics
⇨ Spinal anaesthesia and its complications
⇨ Epidural anaesthesia
⇨ Treatment of bronchial asthma
⇨ Oral hypoglycemia
⇨ Management of diabetes mellitus
⇨ Complications of diabetes mellitus
⇨ Uses of steroids
⇨ Anabolic steroids
⇨ Tocolytics
⇨ Calcium metabolism
⇨ Stages of general anaesthesia
⇨ Preanaesthetic medication.
⇨ Disulfiram
⇨ BZDs
⇨ Treatment of epilepsy
⇨ Lithium carbonate
⇨ Morphine
⇨ Paracitamol poisoning
⇨ Treatment of rheumatoid arthritis
⇨ Digitalis
⇨ Treatment of cardiac arrhythmias
⇨ GTN
⇨ Nifedipine
⇨ Treatment of hypertension
⇨ Various iron preparations

⇨ Treatment of anaemias
⇨ Plasma expanders
⇨ Treatment of peptic ulcer
⇨ Treatment of constipation, diarrhoea
⇨ Indications of use of antimicrobial drugs
⇨ Ciprofloxacin, ofloxacin
⇨ Amoxycillin uses
⇨ Cephalosporins
⇨ Uses and limitations of tetracyclines
⇨ Gentamycin, erythromycin
⇨ Doses and adverse effects of antitubercular drugs
⇨ Local and systemic antifungal drugs
⇨ Antiviral drugs
⇨ Antimalarial drugs
⇨ Cyclophosphamide
⇨ Methotrexate
⇨ 5-FU
⇨ Sunscreens
⇨ Vitamin E.

7. DRUG OF CHOICE

1. Actinomycosis --------------- Penicillin-G (IM)
2. Acute congestive
    glaucoma ---------------------- Pilocarpine nitrate (drops)
3. Acute LVF --------------------- Morphine (IV)
4. Acute severe asthma -------- Aminophylline (IV)
5. Alcohol addiction ----------- Disulfiram
6. Amoebiasis -------------------- Metronidazole (oral)
7. Amoebic liver abscess ------ Metronidazole, emitine,
    chloroquine
8. Anaphylactic shock --------- Adrenaline (SC)
9. Asthma ------------------------ Salbutamol (inhalation),
    Aminophylline
10. Belladonna poisoning ------ Phyostigmine (IV)
11. Brucellosis -------------------- Tetracycline (oral)
12. Burkitt's lymphoma --------- Cyclophosphamide (oral)
13. Campylobacter enteritis ---- Fluoroquinolones
14. Chlamydia -------------------- Tetracycline (oral)
15. Chanceroid -------------------- Cotrimoxazole (oral)
16. CHF ------------------------------ Digoxin (oral)
17. Chronic congestive
    glaucoma ---------------------- Pilocarpine nitrate (topical)
18. Chronic gout ------------------ Probenecid (oral)
19. Chronic gout ------------------ Probenecid (oral) / Allopurinol
20. Chronic myeloid
    leukemia ---------------------- Busulfam (oral)
21. Cirrhotic edema -------------- Spironolactone (oral)
22. Clostridium difficale -------- Vancomycin
23. Cryptococcal meningitis --- Fluconazole
24. Cyanide poisoning ---------- Sodium nitrate (IV)
25. Cystinuria --------------------- Penicillamine
26. Diazepam poisoning ------- Flumazenil (IV)
27. Digitalis induced
    tachycardia -------------------- Phenytoin
28. Diphtheroids ----------------- Vancomycin (IV)
29. Dissociated analgesia ------ Ketamine (IV), Ethylate (IV)
30. Drug induced
    parkinsonism ---------------- Trihexyphenidyl

31. Endogenous depression --- Imipramine, trazodone
32. Endometriosis ---------------- Danazol (oral)
33. Enteric fever -------------------- Ciprofloxacin (oral)
34. Estrogen dependent
    breast cancer ------------------- Tamoxifen
35. Fibrinolysis -------------------- Alteplase (rt-PA) (IV)
36. Filariasis ----------------------- Diethylcarbamazine citrate (oral)
37. Gameticidal -------------------- Primaquine (oral)
38. Genital herpes ---------------- Acyclovir (topical) (oral)
39. Gonorrhoea -------------------- Procaine, penicillin (IM)
40. Gout (acute attack) ---------- NSAID (Indomethacin)
41. Grand mal epilepsy --------- Phenytoin (oral)
42. Guinea worm infestation -- Niridazole (oral)
43. *H. influenzal* meningitis ---- Chloramphenicol (IV)
44. *H. influenzal* pneumonia --- Chloramphenicol (oral)
45. *H. nana* infestation ----------- Praziquantel (oral)
46. *H. simplex*
    keratoconjunctivitis --------- Idoxuridine (topical)
47. Heparin antagonist --------- Protamine sulphate
48. Hg poisoning ------------------ Dimercaprol (IV)
49. Hookworm infestation ----- Pyrantel pamoate (oral), Mebendazole
50. Hydatid disease ------------- Albendazole
51. Hypertensive emergency -- Sodium nitroprusside (IV), GTN (IV), Diazoxide (IV)
52. Insecticide poisoning ------- Pralidoxime and atropine (IV)
53. Iron poisoning --------------- Desferrioxamine
54. Kala azar (resistant) -------- Pentamidine (IM)
55. Legionnaire's pneumonia - Erythromycin (oral)
56. Lepra reaction ---------------- Clofozemine (oral)
57. Listerosis ---------------------- Penicillin-G (IM)
58. Lymphogranuloma
    venerum ----------------------- Tetracycline (oral)
59. Male contraceptives --------- Gossipol (oral)
60. Malignant hyperthermia -- Dentrolene (IV)
61. Mania-depressive ----------- Lithium carbonate (oral)
62. Meningococcal
    pneumonia (prophylaxis) - Rifampicin (oral)

63. Methecillin resistance ------ Vancomycin (IV)
64. Methotrexate poisoning ---- Folinic acid (IV)
65. Methyl alcohol poisoning - 4-methyl pyrazole (IV)
66. Microprolactenemia -------- Bromocriptine
67. Migraine (prophylaxis) ---- Propranolol (oral)
68. Monilial vaginitis ----------- Nystatin (oral)
69. Morphine poisoning -------- Naloxone (IV)
70. Motion sickness -------------- Hyoscine (oral, IV)
71. Myasthenia gravis ---------- Neostigmine (oral)
72. Mycoplasmal pneumonia - Erythromycin (oral)
73. Myxoedema coma ----------- Liothyronine (IV)
74. Nephrogenic diabetes
    Inspidus ---------------------- Thiazide
75. Neurocysticercosis ---------- Praziquantel (oral)
76. Neurogenic diabetes
    mellitus ---------------------- ADH (intranasal)
77. Neurolept analgesia -------- Fentanyl droperidol (IV)
78. Noctural enuresis ----------- Imipramine (oral)
79. Obssessive-compulsive/
    phobic state -------------------- Trazodone (oral)
80. Obstetric local analgesia -- Bupivacaine
81. Organophosphate
    poisoning --------------------- Atropine (IV)
82. Paraoxymal supra-
    ventricular tachycardia ---- Verapamil (IV)
83. Pb poisoning ----------------- Calcium disodium EDTA
84. PCM poisoning -------------- N-acetylcystine (IV),
85. Penicillinase resistance ---- Methecillin (IM/IV)
86. Peptic ulcer -------------------- Omeprazole (oral)
87. Petit mal epilepsy ----------- Ethosuximide (oral)
88. Pneumococcal
    pneumonia -------------------- Penicillin (IM)
89. Pneumocystitis carinii ----- Pentamidine +
                                   Cotrimoxazole (IV)
90. Postmenopausal
    syndrome --------------------- Estrogen (oral)
91. Postpartum hemorrhage --- Methyl ergotamine
92. Radical cure ------------------- Primaquine (oral)
93. Raised intracranial
    pressure ----------------------- Mannitol (IV)

94. Refractory CHF -------------- Amrinone (IV)
95. Relapsing fever -------------- Tetracycline
96. Rheumatic fever -------------- Aspirin (oral)
97. Rheumatoid arthritis ------- NSAID (Aspirin)
98. Roundworm infestation --- Albendazole (oral)
99. Scabies ------------------------ Benzyl benzoate (topical)
100. Schizophrenia ---------------- Chlorpromazine
101. Shigella enteritis ------------- Norfloxacin (oral)
102. Spastic constipation -------- Dietary fibre
103. Strongyloides stercoralis -- Thiabendazole
104. Syphilis ----------------------- Benzathine—Penicillin (IM)
105. Tapeworm infestation ------ Praziquantel (niclosamide)
                                    (oral)
106. Thyrotoxicosis --------------- Carbimazole + Ppt surgery
107. Tobacco amblyopia --------- Hydrocobalamine
108. Transient insomnia --------- Triazolam, Temazepam
109. Trichomonial, vaginitis ---- Metronidazole (oral)
110. Trigeminal neuralgia ------- Carbamazepine (oral)
111. Trypanosomiasis ------------ Pentamidine
112. Tuberculosis ------------------ INH + R + Z + E (oral)
113. Type III hyperlipidemia ---- Gemfibrozil
114. Type IV hyperlipidemia ---- Nicotinic acid (oral)/
                                    Gemfibrozil
115. Type V hyperlipidemia ---- Nicotinic acid (oral)/
                                    Gemfibrozil
116. Ulcerative colitis ------------- Sulfasalazine (oral)
117. Uterine contraceptive ------- Gossypol (oral)
118. Uterine relaxant -------------- Ritodrine (IV), Salbutamol
119. Ventricular Es ---------------- Lidocaine (IV)
120. Ventricular tachycardia ---- Lidocaine (IV)
121. Visceral leishmaniasis ----- Sodium stibogluconate (IM)
122. Whip worm ------------------- Mebendazole/Albendazole
123. Whooping cough ------------ Erythromycin (oral)
124. Wilson's disease ------------- d-penicillamine (oral)
125. Yersenia enterocolitis ------ Cotrimoxazole

| 8. EXPLAIN WHY |

SOME EXAMPLES (SOLVED)

1. **Rationale for combined used of Al hydroxide with Mg hydroxide in antacid gel.**

BECAUSE:

⇨ $Mg(OH)_2$ is laxative and $Al_2(OH)_3$ constipating. Combination annual each others effect and bowel movement is not affected.

⇨ $Mg(OH)_2$ hastens gastric emptying while $Al_2(OH)_3$ decrease gastric emptying. Combination has no effect on gastric emptying.

2. **Mg trisilicate in treatment of peptic ulcer.**

BECAUSE:

⇨ Mg trisilicate produces silica by reacting with HCl. Silica produced is gelatinous, it is absorbed and inactivates pepsin and protects ulcer base by forming coating over it and prevents contact of HCl to ulcer base.

⇨ Has good ANC.

⇨ Does not increases pH more than 3.

3. **ACH is not used therapeutically.**

BECAUSE:

⇨ (i) It is irritant, (ii) Because of evanescent and nonselective action and degrades fastly (t½: 2 to 5 min).

4. **Atropinic drugs also prevent laryngospasm.**

⇨ Atropinic drugs have no action on laryngeal muscles as they are skeletal muscles. Atropinic drugs reduce respiratory secretions that reflexly predispose to laryngospasm and hence prevent laryngospasm.

5. **Ephedrine is orally active while adrenaline is not.**

⇨ Ephedrine is resistant to MAO (monoamine oxidase) so it is not degraded by liver and hence is orally active.

6. **Sch first causes stimulation and then paralysis of skeletal muscles.**

⇨ Sch is a depolarizing blockers and has intrinsic activity for NM receptors. It depolarizes muscle end plate by opening Na^+ channels and initially producing twitching and fasciculations. It does not dissociate rapidly from receptor then all Ach gets depleted and hence causes paralysis.

7. **D-TC causes fill in BP.**

BECAUSE:
⇨ Ganglionic blockade,
⇨ Histamine release and
⇨ Reduces venous return.

8. **Sch in some individual causes prolonged apnoea.**

⇨ Normally pseudocholinesterase breaks Sch into succinic acid and choline. In some individuals pseudocholinesterase is absent hence Sch is not hydrolysed and causes prolonged apnoea by phase II blockade resulting in muscle paralysis and apnoea lasting hours.

9. **Oxethazine is a good anaesthetic for gastric mucosa while other LA are not.**

⇨ Oxethazine is a good, potent topical anaesthetic. It has unique property to ionise to a very small extent even at low pH. It is therefore highly effective in anesthesing gastric mucosa by acting on receptors from inside.

10. **Salbutamol is preferred over isoprenaline in treatment of bronchial asthma.**

BECAUSE:
⇨ Salbutamol is highly β_2 selective whereas isoperaline is $\beta_1 + \beta_2$ selective isoprenaline causes tachycardia via β_1 receptor whereas this disadvantage is not encountered with salbutamol.
⇨ Salbutamol is safer and longer acting than isoprenaline.

11. **Aminophylline is given by slow IV injection.**

⇨ Rapid IV injection of aminophylline causes precordial pain syncope and even sudden death due to marked fall in BP. Ventricular arrhythmias or asystole hence given by slow IV injection.

12. Antihistamines are ineffective in bronchial asthma.

BECAUSE:

⇨ LT and PAF are more important mediators than histamine which are not antagonised by antihistamines.

⇨ Concentration at site may not be sufficient to block high concentration of histamine.

⇨ They do not have bronchodilator action.

13. Halothan causes malignant hyperthermia.

⇨ Due to intracellular release of Ca^{++} from sacroplasmic reticulum causing persistent muscle contraction and increased heat production hence cause malignant hyperthermia.

14. Morphine causes vasodilatation.

BECAUSE:

⇨ Direct action decreases tone of muscles ⎤

⇨ Histamine release ⎟ ↓ BP

⇨ Depression of vasomotor centre. ⎦

15. Neurolept analgesic should not be used in person with parkinsonism.

⇨ In parkinsonism extrapyramidal symptom are due to ↓ in dopamine. Droperidol in neurolept analgesic is a dopamine antagonist it will further aggravate parkinsonism so it is not given in parkinsonism.

16. Antipsychotic drugs are ineffective in motion sickness.

⇨ These drugs act via dopaminergic pathway through CTZ which is not involved in motion sickness. Hence, ineffective in this condition.

EW: Half life of a drug varies for drugs undergoing zero order kinetics (2006)

SN: Polypharmacy (2006)

SN: Drug tolerance (2006)

SN: Pharmacovigilance (2006).

17. Oxazepman used in elderly and in patients with liver disease as antianxiety.

⇨ Its hepatic metabolism is in significant and of short duration of action hence used. Also used in short lasting anxiety cases.

18. **Why there is not antidote for acute barbiturate poisoning.**

⇨ In barbiturate poisoning patient is in comatose. If antidote used in attempt to awaken the patient (e.g. Metrazole) then it is dangerous because it may precipitate convulsion and morbidity and mortality is increased, hence no antidote.

19. **Gastric lavage is done in morphine poisoning even if drug is injected.**

⇨ Morphine is a basic drug, it is partitioned to gastric acid juice. To prevent its diffusion back into blood gastric lavage is done with $KMnO_4$.

20. **Morphine is contraindicated in bronchial asthma.**

BECAUSE:

⇨ Morphine can precipitate attack of bronchial asthma by histamine release

⇨ It depresses respiratory and cough centre, hence contraindicated.

21. **Overdose of pathidine produces many excitatory effects while it is equally sedative as morphine.**

⇨ In overdose of pathidine, its metabolite norphathidine accumulates which has excitatory action.

22. **Why morphine is used in acute left ventricular failure.**

BECAUSE:

⇨ It decreases preload on heart by causing peripheral pooling of blood.

⇨ It tends to shift blood from pulmonary to systemic circulation.

⇨ It calms air hunger by causing respiratory depression.

⇨ It cuts sympathetic innervation by calming the patient → Reduces cardiac work.

23. **Aspirin causes gastric bleeding.**

⇨ It is a acidic drug and remains unionised and diffusible in gastric acid juice → enters mucosal cell and ionise and become indiffusible (ion trapping).

⇨ Further aspirin particles coming in contract with gastric mucosa promote local back diffusion of acid → focal necrosis of mucosal cells → acute ulcers, erosive gastritis, congestion and microscopic bleeding → gastric bleeding.

24. PCM has no anti-inflammatory property.

⇨ At the site of inflammation peroxidase is formed, which inhibits PCM and hence it is not able to inhibits cox in presence of peroxidase → no anti-inflammatory property.

25. KCl is given in diabetic ketoacidosis.

⇨ K^+ is lost in urine during ketoacidosis and serum K^+ is usually normal due to exchange with intracellular stores when insulin therapy is started, ketoacidosis subsides and K^+ is driven intracellular → dangerous hypokalemic can occur hence KCl is given in diabetic ketoacidosis.

26. Biguanides not used in underweight patients with NIDDM.

⇨ They have anorectic action and can further reduce weight and complications may appear so not given in underweight patients with NIDDM. Biguanides also inhibit intestinal absorption of glucose, amino acids and vitamin B_{12}.

27. Progesterone is added to estrogen in OC while later alone can promote contraception.

BECAUSE:

⇨ Progesterone ensure prompt bleeding at the end of cycle and blocks the risk of developing endometrial carcinoma due to estrogen hence it is added with estrogen.

⇨ Both estrogen and progesterone synergist to inhibit ovulation.

28. Estrogen in high doses is effective as post-coital contraception.

⇨ High dose of estrogen with or without progesterone given for few days and then discontinued induces bleeding → the postcoital pill may thus dislodge a just implanted blastocyst or may interfere with fertilization or implantation.

29. Estrogen is favourable to sperm penetration.

BECAUSE:

⇨ Increase rhythmic contraction of fallopian tubes and uterus.

⇨ Induces a watery secretion from cervix.

30. **Estrogen component of OC is mainly responsible for venous thromboembolism.**

BECASUE:
- ➪ Increase blood coagulation factors,
- ➪ Decrease antithrombin III
- ➪ Decrease plasminogen activator in endothelium, and
- ➪ Increase platelet aggregation.

31. **Oxytocin is given by slow IV infusion and in low doses.**

BECASUE:
- ➪ Because of its shorter t½ and slow IV infusion, intensity of action can be controlled and action can be quickly terminated.
- ➪ Low concentrate allow Normal relaxations between contraction → foetal oxygenation does not suffer.
- ➪ Lower segment is not contracted → foetal descent is not compromised.

32. **Ergotamine and methyl ergotamine are preferred over oxytocin to stop bleeding.**

- ➪ Because they cause sustained tonic contraction → the perforating arteries are compressed by myometrial mesh work → bleeding stops which is not achieved by oxytocin. Hence preferred over oxytocin.

33. **Estrogen is contraindicated during pregnancy.**

BECASUE:
- ➪ It increases incidence of vaginal cancer is ? offspring.
- ➪ Increases incidences of genital abnormalities in ? offspring.
Hence it is contraindicated in pregnancy.

34. **Caffeine and ergotamine are given in migraine.**

BECASUE:
- ➪ Caffeine constricts cerebral vessels → reduces headache.
- ➪ Caffeine ↑es absorption of ergotemine.
- ➪ They act synergistically.

35. **Doxycycline is safest in renal failure.**

BECASUE:
- ➪ Ninety percent drug is excreted in feces as conjugated.
- ➪ t½ is not affected by renal failure.
- ➪ It does not aggravate azootemia.
- ➪ Higher levels are maintained longer → less toxicity.

36. **Tetracycline should not be given to children.**

BECAUSE:

⇨ It has antianabolic effect.

⇨ Tetracycline forms orthophosphate complex which gets deposited in developing bones and teeth and cause brown discoloration of teeth.

⇨ Defective enamel causes hypoplasia of teeth.

⇨ Increases risk of caries.

37. **Tetracycline should not be given to pregnant women.**

⇨ Because it crosses placenta and temporarily suppresses bone gowth → retardation of fetal bone growth and it also causes ↑ in intracranial pressure in some infants.

38. **Penicillin is not toxic to man but is toxic to microorganism.**

⇨ Penicillin inhibits peptidoglycan cell wall synthesis and human beings have no cell wall. Also it is needed in low concentration hence not toxic to man.

39. **Tetracycline is not given in sore throat.**

BECAUSE:

⇨ Sore throat is usually viral in origin where it is ineffective.

⇨ Resistance develops and it is also costly and other more effective antibiotics are available.

40. **NaHCO$_3$ is not the antacid of choice.**

BECAUSE:

⇨ In the intestine it is unable to neutralize HCO$_3^-$ and hence causes systemic alkalosis.

⇨ Short duration of action.

⇨ ↑es pH >2.5 and hence impair digestion.

⇨ Produces CO$_2$ in stomach → abdominal discomfort.

⇨ It may worsen CHF and edema by ↑ing Na$^+$ load.

9. DOSES OF SOME IMPORTANT DRUGS IN CHILDREN

Method of calculation of drug dose in children in general, Clark's rule is applicable if adult dose is known

1. Dose in children = $\dfrac{\text{Wt of child in lbs}}{150}$ × Adult dose.

2. $\dfrac{SA}{1.7}$ × Adult dose

3. SA of child in M2 × 60 = % of Adult dose.

A. ANALGESICS, ANTIPYRETICS AND ANTI-INFLAMMATORY DRUGS

1. Acetylsalicylic acid—30-65 mg/kg/day 6 hr oral
2. Codeine phosphate—3 mg/kg/day qid
3. Dextropropoxyphane hydrochloride—2-4 mg/kg/day bd
4. Diclopherol Na—2-5 mg/kg/day tds
5. Ibuprofen—20 mg/kg/day tds
6. Indomethacin—3 mg/kg/day tds
7. Morphine SO_4—0.1-0.2 mg/kg/day SC
8. Nimesulide—5 mg/kg 8-12 hr
9. Paracetamol—30-60 mg/kg/day 4-6 hr oral
   or 10 mg/kg/day injection
   or injection 5 mg/kg/day single dose
10. Pethidine hydrochloride—1-2 mg/kg/dose IM or IV.

B. ANTHELMINTICS

1. Albendazole—200 mg single dose (1-2 yrs)
   400 mg > 2 yrs children and adult.
2. Levamisol—2 mg/kg single dose at night for ascariasis.
3. Mebendazole—100 mg bd × 3 days for ascariasis
   200 mg bd × 3 days for tapeworms repeat after 2 weeks
   for hydatid cyst—30 mg/kg/day 8 hrly oral × 4 weeks
4. Niclosamide—1 gm empty stomach followed by next dose after 1 hr
5. Parziquntel—50 mg/kg/day 8 hrly oral × 10-14 days
6. Pyrantel pamoate—11 mg/kg single dose

C. ANTIBIOTIC AND CHEMOTHERAPEUTIC AGENTS

1. Aminoglycosides
   A. Amikacin*—7.5 mg/kg/dose IV/IM
   B. Gentamycin sulfate*—2.5 mg/kg/dose IM/IV
   C. Kanamycin sulfate*—2.5 mg/kg/dose IM/IV
   D. Neomycin sulfate—12.5 mg/kg/dose oral in diarrhea and 3 g/m^2/day 6 hrly in hepatic coma
   E. Streptomycin—30-40 mg/kg/day 12 hrly.
      * every 12 hr for infants below 0-7 days and 8 hrly for infants > 7 days.

D. CEPHALOSPORINS

1. Cefadroxil—15 mg/kg/dose 12 hr oral
2. Cefazolin Na—20 mg/kg/dose IM IV
   IV should be given over 15-20 min
3. Cefixime—8 mg/kg/dose oran once or twice
4. Cefotaxime Na—50 mg/kg/dose
5. Ceftazidime—50 mg/kg/dose IM IV
6. Ceftriaxone Na—50-75 mg/kg/dose
7. Cephlexin—7-12 mg/kg/dose 6 hr orally.

E. LINCOSAMIDES

A. Clindamycin hydrochloride
   0-7 days—5 mg/kg/dose 8 hr oral IV
   > 7 days—5 mg/kg/dose 6 hrly
B. Lincomycin hydrochloride
   5-10 mg/kg/dose 12 hrly IM IV

F. MACROLIDES

A. Azithromycin dihydrate—10 mg/kg/day single dose empty stomach × 3 days
B. Erythromycin—5-12.5 mg/kg/dose 6-8 hrly
   5 mg/kg/dose IV as infusion over 8 hr with normal saline or Ringer lactate
C. Roxythromycin—2.5 mg/kg/dose 12 hrly.

G. PENICILLINS

1. Amoxicillin—25-50 mg/kg/day 8 hr orally

2. Ampicillin with salbutam—150 mg/kg/day 8 hr IM or IV
   Cotanin 100 mg ampicillin/50 mg salbactum
3. Cloxacillin*—12.5 mg/kg/dose oral or IV
4. Methicillin Na*—25 mg/kg/dose
5. Penicillin G (aquous)*—25,000 units/kg/dose IM IV.
   * Preterm infants = upto 70 mg—every 12 hrly
   Term upto 7 days—8 hrly
   and preterm infant > 2 days
   and term baby > 7 days—6 hrly

H. SULPHAS

1. Sulphonamide—100-150 kg/day 8 hrs oral
2. Timethoprim + Sulfamethoxazole (Cotrimoxazole)
   Neonates—2 mg/kg/days loading dose followed by 1.2 mg/kg/day 12 hrly
   Children—5-8 mg/kg or TMP or 25-50 mg/kg of SM2/day 12 hrly oral.

I. MISCELLANEOUS ANTIMICROBIALS

1. Chloramphenicol—25 mg/kg/dose oral IM IV
2. Ciprofloxacin—5-10 mg/kg/dose 12 hr
   avoide in children < 12 years because of cartilage toxicity
3. Furazolidine—2 mg/kg/dose every 6-8 hr
4. Nalidixic acid—50 mg/kg/day 6-8 hr oral
5. Norfloxacin—7.5-10 mg/kg/day 12 hr oral
6. Ofloxacin—7.5 mg/kg/day
   IV dose—5 mg/kg/dose 12 hrly
7. Tetracycline hydrochloride—3-6 mg/kg/dose 6 hr oral
   + Avoid children < 8 years.

J. ANTICONVULSANTS

1. Carbamazepine—10-20 mg/kg/day 8 hr oral
   less than 1 year 200 mg
   1-5 years—400 mg
   5-10 years—600 mg
   > 10 years 800-100 mg.
2. Clonazepam—0.02 mg/kg/day 12 hrly oral
3. Diazepam—0.2-0.3 mg/kg/dose
4. Ethosuximide—20-70 mg/kg/day 12 hrly

5. Phenobarbitone Na—3-10 mg/kg/day or single dose at night 12 hours oral
6. Phenytoin sodium—4-12 mg/kg/day 12 hrly or single oral dose
7. Prednisolone—2 mg/kg/day 8 hrly for 2-6 hours
8. Valproate Na—15 mg/kg/day 8-12 hrly orally.

K. ANTIEMETICS

1. Domperidone—0.2-0.4 mg/kg/dose 4-8 hrly
2. Metochlorpromide HCl—0.1 mg/kg/day 6-8 hr oral or IM
3. Ondansetron HCL dihydrate—5 mg/m^2 IV prior to procedure followed by 4 mg oral × bd × 5 days
4. Triflupromazine—0.5 mg/kg/day 8 hr oral.

L. ANTIHISTAMINES

1. Astemizole—0.2-1 mg/kg/dose singl dose oral
2. Cetrizine dihydrochloride
   5 mg for < 30kg
   10 mg > 30 kg oral od
3. Chlorphenamine maleate—0.5 mg/kg/dose 8 hr oral.

M. ANTIHYPERTENSIVES

1. Atenolol—1-2 mg/kg/dose single dose
2. Captopril—3 mg/kg/dose 8 hrly
3. Methyldopa—10-40 mg/kg/dose 8-12 hrly
4. Nifedipine—0.5-1 mg/kg/dose 8 hrly oral
5. Propranolol 2-4 mg/kg/dose 8 hrly oral
6. Na nitroprusside—0.5 to 8 mcg/kg/mt
7. Verapamil—2-4 mg/kg/dose 8 hrly oral.

N. ANTILEPROTIC

1. Clofazime—1-2 mg/kg/daily and
   4-6 mg/kg once a month
2. Diaminodiphenyl sulphone (DDS)—1-2 mg/kg/dose.

O. ANTIMALARIAL DRUGS

1. Chloroquine PO4—10 mg of base/kg state followed 5 mg/kg 6 hr later and once a day oral × 2 hrly
2. Mefloquine—15-25 mg/kg/single dose
3. Quinine sulphate—25 mg/kg/day 8 hrly × 7 days.

P. ANTITUBERCULAR (ANTI-TB)

1. Isoniazid—5-10 mg/kg/day single dose
2. Rifampicin—10 mg/kg/day single dose empty 8 hrly
3. Pyrazinamide—20-35 mg/kg/day single dose
4. Ethambutol—25 mg/kg/day single dose oral × 4 weeks
   then 15 mg/kg/hrly
   Streptomycin sulfate—20-40 mg/kg/day IM daily.

Q. MISCELLANEOUS DRUGS

1. Adrenaline—0.01 ml/kg/dose of 1:1000 solution SC.
2. Aminophyline—15-20 mg/kg/dose 8 hrly oral
   For status asthmatics—5-7 mg/kg loading dose IV followed
   by 0.09 mg/kg/hr.
3. Metronidazole—15-20 mg/kg 8 hrly oral and 20 mg/kg/
   dose 8 hrly IV for anaerobic infant
4. Human hepatitis B specific globulins—0.06-0.1 ml/kg IM at
   the time of exposure
5. Tetanus antitoxins
   Prophylactic—3,000-5,000 units SC 1 hrly
   Therapeutics—10,000 units IM IV.
6. Salbutamol—0.1-0.4 mg/kg/dose 8 hrly
7. Digoxin—Digitalizing dose
   Premature—0.04 mg/kg/day
   Full term—0.06 mg/kg/day
   < 2 years children—0.06 mg/kg/day
   > 2 year children—0.04 mg/kg/day oral
   The daily maintenance digoxin is about 1/4 of initial
   digitalizing dose.
8. Furosamide—2-4 mg/kg/day 12 hrly oral
   IV dose is 1.2 of oral dose
9. Lithium carbonate—10-15 mg/kg/day 8 hrly oral to maintain
   blood 1 eml b/w—0.75 to 1 mEq/l.
10. Ranitidine—2-4 mg/kg/day 12 hrly.

10. IMPORTANT POINTS

⇨ Potency of the drug refers to the **amount of drug** needed to produce a given response.

⇨ Efficacy of the drug refers o the **maximal response** that can be produced by the drug.

⇨ ED_{50} is the dose of drug required to produce 50% of the maximum response. It is a measure of potency of drug.

⇨ Zero order kinetics = rate of elimination = constant, CL ↓ with ↑ in concentration of drug.
  - Ethyl alcohol
  - Tolbutamide
  - Theophylline
  - Propanolol   } Follow the zero order kinetics
  - Phenytoin
  - Warfarin
  - Aspirin

⇨ First order kinetics = Rate of elimination is directly proportional to concentration of the drug.
  CL remains constant.

⇨ Uses of microsomal enzyme induction:
  1. Cong. Nonhemolytic jaundice (phenobarbitone)
  2. Cushing's syndrome = Phenytoin may reduce the manifestation.
  3. Chronic poisonings
  4. Liver disease

⇨ Therapeutic index = Safty margin = $\dfrac{LD50}{ED50} = \dfrac{Med.\,ethal\,dose}{Med.\,effective\,dose}$

⇨ Bioavailability is a measure of fraction of administered dose of a drug that reactes the systemic circulation in the unchanged form (100% of drug injected IV)

⇨ Steroid hormones act on cytoplasmic receptor → nucleus, thyroid hormones act on nuclear reception while others act on cell membrane receptors.

⇨ National essential drug list (1996) = 279 drugs included.

⇨ P-450 enzyme inhibitors:
  - Ciprofloxacin
  - Omeprazole
  - Metronidazole
  - Erythromycin
  - Ketoconazole
  - Cimetidine

⇨ Autonomic drugs = $\begin{cases} \text{Acetylcholine, muscarine} \\ \text{Methacholine, pilocarpine} \end{cases}$

= produce actions similar to Acetylcholine

⇨ Anticholinesterases (Anti Ches) = (-) Che thus protects the Acetylcholine from hydrolysis = produce cholinergic effects and potentiates Acetylcholine

- Physostigmine ⎤
- Edrophonium   ⎬ Reversible
- Neostigmine   ⎟
- Tacrine   ⎦

- Melathion   ⎤
- Parathione ⎟
- Tabun   ⎬ Irreversible
- Carbaryl   ⎟
- Propoxur   ⎦

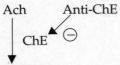

Ach   Anti-ChE

ChE ⊖

Breakdown

⇨ Anticholinergic drugs = block actions of Ach on ANS and act via muscarinic receptors in CNS.
  - Atropine
  - Hyosine
  - Homatropine
  - Ipratropium bromide
  - Cyclopentolate
  - Tropicamide
  - Glycopyrolate
  - Pirenzepine
  - Telenzepine
  - Benzhexol (trihexy phenidyl).

⇨ Pralidoxime (2-PAM) = in Anti-cholinesterase poisoning (organophosphorus poisoning) (also atropins) 2 mg IV till pupil dialates at an interval of 10 min. upto 200 mg in one day)

⇨ First line antitubercular drugs are tuberculocidal except ethambutol

⇨ 2nd line drugs are tuberculostatic
⇨ Other uses of rifampin
1. Leprosy
2. Systemic fungal infection with amphotericin B)
3. Prophylaxis of meningococcal meningitis
4. Legionella infection
5. Brucellosis (with doxycyclins).

⇨ **Side effect of various ATT drugs.**

1. Arthralgia = INH and pyrazinamide
2. Hyperuricemia = ethambutol, pyrazinamide
3. Optic neuritis = isoniazid, Ethambutol
4. Hepatitis = Inn, rifampicin, pyrazinamide
5. Peripheral neuropathy = Streptomycin INH, Ethambutol, ethionamide
6. Ototoxicity and renal toxicity = Streptomycin (CI in pregnancy)
7. Pigmentation = Rifampicin
8. Cataract, red green colour blindness ethambutol
9. Neutrosychiatric manifestation = Cycloserine

Thiazetaxone is CI in AIDS patients.

⇨ **Treatment of TB in pregnanacy**

• INH + Rifampicin = 9 months
  Add E if resistance to INH suspected
• Pyridoxine 50 mg daily
• It should cover delivery and perpeuriam
• In case of active lesion T should continuous 6 months following delivery or until the disease is amsted
⇨ Effective ATT reduces infectively upto 90% in 48 hours.

⇨ **Drug and their mechanism of action.**

1. Inhibition of cell wall synthesis ← inhibition of mycolic acid synthesis ← Isoniazid (INH)
   = Penicillins, cephalosporins
   Cycloserine, vancomycin, bacitracin

2. Inhibition of protein synthesis ◄─────────────────┐

- Tetra-   • Clinda-   • Aminoglycoside → Misreading of
  cycline   mycin   • Streptomycin   m RNA code
- Chloram- • Mupirocin
  phenicol
- Erythro- • Griseofulvin
  mycin

3. Interfere with intermediatory metabolism
   = Sulfonamides, trimethoprim, ethambutol, PAS
4. Inhibition of nucleic acid synthesis
   = Quinolines, flucyosine, rifampin
5. Inhibition of HMG GA reductase
   = Lovastatin, merastatin, simvastatin.

⇨ **Drugs causing gynaecomastia:**

- Calcium channel blockers
- Digitalis
- Ketoconazole
- Griseofulvin
- INH
- Ethionamide
- Estrogen
- Testosterone
- Methyldopa
- Phenytoin
- Reserpine
- Cimetidine
- Amiodarone
- Clomiphine.

⇨ **Agents inducing theophylline metabolism**
   (↓ its plasma level, toxicity)

- Rifampicin
- Phenytoin
- Phenobarbitone
- Smoking

⇨ **Agents which inhibit theophyline metabolism**
(enhance toxicity)
- Erythromycin
- Ciprofloxacin
- Oral contraceptives
- Cimetidine
- Allopurinol.

⇨ PCM produces highly reactive toxic minor metabolite = N-acetyl benzoquinone amine Antidote = N-acetyl cystine.

⇨ Lipid insoluble alpha blockers (do not cross BBB)
Atenolol
Nadolol
Sotalol = Excreted in urine so should not be used in renal failure.

⇨ Septran (TMP-SMI) is Doc for:
- Moraxella catarrhalis
- Haemophilus
- Nocardia
- Enterobacter
- Wipple's disease = T. septran 1 bd (DS) × 1yr

⇨ Penicillin G is Metabolized by kidney (mainly)
    < 10% is eliminated by glomerular filtration.
    90% is eliminated by tubular secretion

⇨ DOC for PSVT = Adenosine (2nd verapamil)

⇨ Red man Syndrome = Pruritis, flushing, erythema of head and upper toxo = Caused by vancomycin

⇨ Drug raising intracranial pressure:
Steroids, hypervitaminosis A, oral contraceptive, tetracyclines amiodarone, quinolones.

⇨ Oral anticoagulants act by interfering with prothrombin, factor VII, IX, X

⇨ Non-selective α blockers = Ergotamine, Dihydroxyergotamine (DHE) chlorpromazine phentolamine, ergotamine

⇨ Non-selective β blockers = $(\beta_1 + \beta_2)$ = Propranolol, sotalol, Timolol, oxprenolol
Labetalol and Carvedilol = with α blocking property = (α + β blocker)

⇨ β_1 blocker (cardioselective)
Atenolol, Metoprolol, Esmolol, Betaxolol, Bisoprolol

⇨ Bone marrow suppression is the most serious toxicity of anticancer drugs with often limits the dose. Infections and bleeding are usual complications.

Anticancer drug	*Prominant side effects*
1. Actinomycin D	Alopecia, BMS
2. Bleomycin	Pulmonary fibrosis
3. Busulphan	Pulmonary fibrosis, hyperuricemia
4. Cyclophosphamide	Alopecia, hemorrhagic cystitis
5. Doxorubicin	Cardiotoxicity
6. Methotrexate	BMS, acute renal failure, Histotoxicity
7. Vincristine	Alopecia, Peripheral neuropathy
8. Melphalan	Pulmonary fibrosis

➪ ACE inhibitors and angiotensin antagonists (Losartan) are contraindicated in pregnancy.

➪ T_3 & T_4
1. Thyroid secretes more T_4 than T_3
2. T_4 = More tightly bound to plasma protein (15 times) = major circulatory hormone
3. T_3 = 5 times more potent than T_4
4. 1/3rd of T_4 is converted T_3 is in peripheral tissues
5. T_3 is more avidely bound to nuclear receptors than T_4

➪ Diabetic ketoacidosis treatment =
• Insulin
• IV fluid = to combat dehydration
• KCl = to prevent hypokalemia as K^+ is driven intracellularlly with insulins therapy)
• Sodium bicarbonate = if pH < 7.1
• Antibiotics
• Phosphate

➪ Indications of purer/human insulins:
1. Insulin resistance
2. Allergy to conventional preparations
3. Injection site lipodystrophy
4. Short-term of insulin (Diabetic)
5. Pregnancy

➪ Uterine
- Stimulants = Oxytocin, ergotamine, misoprostol
- Relaxants = Salbutamol, terbuline, Mg^{++} Salts, CCBs C_2H_5OH, PG synthesis inhibitors

⇨ Edrophonium 2 mg IV $\Big\langle$ Improvement = "Myasthenia gravis"

Worsening = cholinergic crisis.

⇨ 1.5 mg neostigmine (IM) = improve = "Myasthenia gravis"

⇨ Side effects of phenytoin = Megaloblastic Anaemia, osteomalacia, Pancytopenias and H^5 = Hypertrophy of gums, Hirsutism, hyperglycemia, hypersensitivity hydantoin Syndrome.

⇨ Side effect of cisplatin = vomiting

⇨ Side effect of cisapride = Diarrhoeas

⇨ Tamsulosin = α_1 A antagonist (DYNAPRESS)

⇨ +ve intopic action = ↑ in force of contraction (↑ myocardial contractibility)

⇨ Erythromycin:

Treatment of choice in:
–   Pertusis
–   Mycoplasma pneumonia infection
–   Legionnaire's disease (Azithromycin)
–   Diphtheria carriers → erythrasma
–   Chancroid

⇨ Treatment of choice of cholera
1. *Adults:* Doxycycline 300 mg single dose = DOC (or tetracycline 500 mg tid × 3d)
2. *Children:* Septran (Sulfamethoxazole + Trimethoprim)
3. *Pregnant women:* Furazolidine 100 mg q id × 3d

⇨ 5HT receptor

• 5HT1: $\Big\langle$ 5HT1A = Buspirone (agonist)

5HT1D = Sumatriptan (Agonist)

• 5HT2: 5HT2A = Ketanserine, cyproheptadine (Antagonists)
• 5HT3 : Ondensetron (Antagonist)
• 5HT4 : Cisapride (Agonist)

MICROBIOLOGY

1. PATTERN OF EXAMINATION

MICROBIOLOGY	Marks
☞ Theory Paper I	40
☞ Theory Paper II	40
☞ Internal Assessment (Theory)	15
☞ Internal Assessment (Prac)	15
☞ Spotting (5 spots)	5
☞ Gram's Stain	5
☞ Stool Examination	5
☞ Clinical Problem	5
☞ Special Stain	5
☞ Theory Viva	15
Total	150

*Note:*Every theory paper comperises of 8 short notes of 5 marks each.

Paper I =   *   General Microbiology
         *   Immunology
         *   Bacteriology
Paper II =   *   Virology
         *   Parasitology
         *   Mycology

2. QUESTIONS FOR THEORY PAPER

A. GENERAL MICROBIOLOGY

SN: Write briefly on bacterial cell wall (2004)

SN: Bacterial growth curve

LQ: Name the various methods of gene transfer and describe briefly about "conjugation" (2005)

DW: Fungal and bacterial cell (2000)

SN: Draw a bacterial growth curve. Write briefly on its various phases (1998)

SN: L form of bacteria (1993)

SN: Koch's pastulates (1996)

SN: Causative agents of food poisoning

SN: Louis pasteur (1991)

SN: Lysogenic conversion (2000)

SN: Mechanism of transmission of drug resistance in bacteria (2001)

SN: Bacterial capsule (2000)

SN: Working principle and uses of fluorescent microscope in diagnostic microbiology (1997)

SN: Difference between exotoxins and endotoxins (2004)

SN: Autoclave (1998)

SN: Sterilization by moist heat (2001)

SN: Sterilization of heat sensitive surgical equipments (1997)

SN: Bacterial filters (1987)

SN: Exotoxins (2000)

SN: Endotoxins (1994)

SN: Gram's stain (1993)

SN: Negative staining (2000)

SN: Exotoxins and endotoxins

SN: Bacterial plasmids

SN: Bacterial spore (2001)

SN: Discuss spread of drug resistance in bacteria.

SN: Mechanism of transmissible drug resistance in bacteria (1990)

SN: Principles and application of autoclave

SN: Chemical methods of sterilization (2002)

SN: Sterilization by filtration (1993)

SN: Fumigation of operation theatre (1994)

SN: Write the principle and application of sterilization by steam under pressure (1996)

SN: Selective media (1992)

SN: Transport media (1986)

SN: Classify anaerobic bacteria and describe the methods of its cultivation in laboratory (1989)

SN: Anaerobic culture methods

SN: Methods of anaerobiosis (1989)

SN: Plasmid (1995)

SN: Conjugation (1997)

SN: RTF (Resistance transfer factor (1987)

SN: Transduction (1993)

SN: Anaerobic method for bacterial culture (2002)

Que: What is DNA probe? How can it be used in diagnosis of infectious diseases? (1999)

Que: Define plasmids and describe transmission of plasmids among bacteria along with their application in drug resistance (2006)

SN: Bacterial capsule (2006)

Que: Describe briefly principle and functions of hot air oven (2007)

Que: Describe the bacterial growth curve (2008)

LQ: Describe the laboratory diagnosis of anaerobic infections (2008).

B. IMMUNOLOGY

SN: Cell mediated immunity (2005)
SN: Active and passive immunity (1986)
SN: Toxoid (1987)
SN: Immunoglobulin A (2005)
SN: Difference between T cells and B cells (1989)
SN: Identification of T cells and B cells (1986)
SN: Role of thymus in immune response (1992)
SN: T-lymphocytes (1995)
SN: Functions of T lymphocytes (2002)
SN: Adjuvants (1990)
SN: Lymphokines
SN: Monoclonal antibodies (2001)
SN: Monoclonal antibodies and their application
SN: Theories of antibody production
SN: IgE in parasitic infections (1999)
SN: IgM (1997)
SN: Secretory IgA
SN: Structure and properties of IgG
SN: Immunoglobulin G (2004)
SN: Interleukins (2001)
SN: ELISA and its applications (1996)
SN: Immunoelectrophoresis
SN: Indirect fluorescent antibody test (2001)
SN: Principles and application of immunofluorescence test
SN: Radioimmunoassay (1986)
SN: Type- III hypersensitivity (1991)
SN: Classical complement pathway and its biological effects (1989)
SN: Complement (1990)
SN: Complement cascade (1996)
SN: Anaphylactic shock
SN: Type-I hypersensitivity reaction (2001)
SN: Anaphylaxis.(1986)
SN: Type-I hypersensitivity (2002)
SN: Atophy
SN: Delayed hypersensitivity (1983)
SN: Serum sickness (1989)
SN: Immune complex diseases

SN: Allograft (1988)
SN: Graft vs host reaction (1990)
SN: Precipitation reaction
SN: Complement fixation test
SN: Hemolytic disease of the newborn
SN: Local immunity (2000)
SN: Alternate compliment pathway (2001)
SN: Interleukin-2 (2001)
SN: Arthrus reaction (1994)
SN: Western Blot assay (1993)
SN: Antigen receptors on T-lymphocytes (2006)
SN: IgM antibody (2007)
SN: Adjuvants (2007)
SN: Classical complement pathway (2008)
SN: Monoclonal antibodies (2008).

C. BACTERIOLOGY

LQ: Discuss briefly the laboratory diagnosis of diphtheria (2005)

SN: Staphylococcal toxins (1990)

SN: Coagulase test

SN: Coagglutination

LQ: Write briefly on methicillin resistant staphylococcus aureus (MRSA) (2004)

SN: Describe briefly toxic shock syndrome (1995)

LQ: Streptococcal sore throat

LQ: Classify genus streptococcus. Enumerate various lesions produces by group A streptococci (1995)

SN: ASLO test (1994)

SN: Toxins and enzymes of group A streptococci

SN: Describe briefly principle and applications of ASLO test

SN: *Haemophilus influenzae* (2004)

SN: Group B streptococci

SN: Classification of genus streptococci and toxins and enzymes produced by group A streptococci

SN: Acute case of gonorrhoea

LD: Gonorrhoea (1999)

LD: Meningococcal meningitis

LD: Pathogenic meningitis

LQ: Describe laboratory diagnosis of diphtheria (2004)

LD: Purulent meningitis

LQ: Enumerate the etiological agents of pyogenic meningitis. Write laboratory diagnosis of meningococcal meningitis (1993)

LQ: Name various etiological agents of acute pyogenic meningitis. Discuss in detail its laboratory diagnosis (1996)

LQ: Name various etiological agents of sexually transmitted diseases. Describe laboratory diagnosis of gonorrhoea (1995)

LQ: Describe the morphology and growth characters of Corynebacterium diphtheriae

SN: The toxigenicity tests for Corynebacterium diphtheriae

LD: Urinary tract infection

SN: Classification and pathogenesis of genus shigella

SN: *Mycoplasma pneumoniae* (2004)

LD: Salmonella food poisoning

LD: Enteric fever

LD: Enteric fever during the first week

LD: Typhoid carrier

SN: Widal test (1999)

LD: A case of cholera

SN: Enterotoxigenic Escherichia coli (ETEC) (2005)

LD: Cholera

LQ: Describe the morphological and cultural characters of vibrio cholera and differentiate between classical and Eltor vibrio (2000)

SN: Eltor vibrio

LD: Brucellosis

LQ: Classify spirochetes. Enumerate the serological tests for diagnosis of syphilis. Discuss the merits and demerits of each test (2002)

SM   BCG vaccine

SN: Describe any one method of concentration of sputum for culture of *M.tuberculosis*. Classify genus mycobacterium.

SN: Differentiate between *Mycobacterium tuberculosis* and atypical mycobacteria (1994)

SN: The concentration techniques of sputum for the isolation of tubercle bacilli

LQ: Enumerate the causative agents of purulent meningitis. Describe briefly the laboratory diagnosis of such a case (2002)

SN: Clue cells (2000)

SN: Principle and uses of tuberculin test (1989)

SN: Lepromin test (1992)

SN: Name two animal models used to study *Mycobacterium leprae*. Describe the principle method and significance of lepromin test (1995)

LD: Diagnosis of secondary syphilis (1988)

LD: Secondary syphilis.

LQ: Write briefly on Revised National Tuberculosis Control Programme. (RNTCP) (2005)

LD: Specific serological tests for syphilis. Enumerate their advantages and disadvantages

LQ: Classify spirochetes. Enumerate serological tests of syphilis and discuss merits and demerits of each test (2001)

LQ: List the microbes that are associated with sexually transmitted diseases. Write briefly on laboratory diagnosis of syphilis. (2001)

SN: *Mycoplasma pneumonia*

SN: Weil Felix test (1997)

LD: Conjunctivitis

SN: *Chlamydia trachomatis* (1989)

SN: Classify chlamydia and enumerate the disease produced by them

LQ: Name the disease spread through water. Describe bacteriological examination of water

SN: Atypical mycobacteria (2002)

Que: Why penicillin cannot be used to treat *Mycoplasma pneumoniae* infections? (2000)

Que: What is the pathogenesis of most rickettsial diseases (except Q fever)? Why do they cause rash? (2002)

SN: Concentration techniques of sputum for mycobacteria (1993)

Que: Describe laboratory diagnosis of secondary syphilis (2006)

Que: Discuss briefly laboratory Diagnosis of meningitis caused by Haemophilus influenzae (2006)

Que: Discuss briefly Enterotoxigenic Escherichia coli (2006)

SN: Methods of toxin detection of Corynebacterium dephtheriae (2006)

Que: Classify mycobacteria. Write briefly about the laboratory diagnosis of pulmonary tuberculosis (2007)

SN: TRIC agents (2007)

SN: *Helicobacter pylori* (2007)

SN: The pathogenesis of acute rheumatic fever (2008)

SN: Laboratory diagnosis of primary syphilis (2008).

D. VIROLOGY

SN: Polio vaccine (2005)
SN: Interferon (1994)
SN: MMR vaccine (2002)
SN: Pulse Polio Immunisation (2004)
SN: Principle and application of polymerase chain reaction (2002)
SN: Hepatitis B (2004)
SN: Hepatitis B vaccines
SN: Hepatitis B virus and antibodies
SN: Lysogeny
SN: Japanese B encephalitis 1996)
LQ: Enumerate arboviruses. Describe laboratory diagnosis of dengue fever (2004)
SN: Inclusion bodies (1986)
SN: Cultivation of viruses in chick embryo
SN: Rabies vaccines (2000)
LD: Hepatitis B infection
SN: Hepatitis A virus
SN: Name polio vaccines. Discuss their advantages and disadvantages
SN: KD (Kyasanur Forest) disease (1988)
LD: Rabies
SN: Negri body (2001)
SN: Congenital viral infections (2005)
SN: Cultivation of viruses in laboratory (1989)
LQ: Briefly describe the methods by which growth of a virus in cell culture can be identified (2001)
SN: Write about the polio vaccines and the Pulse Polio Programme (2002)
SN: Egg inovulation techniques (1995)
SN: *In vitro* cultivation of viruses
SN: Ebola virus (1996)
SN: Viruses causing diarrhoea in children and laboratory diagnosis of Rota virus diarrhea
SN: Viruses causing human cancer (1997)
SN: Dengue fever (1998)
LD: AIDS
LQ: Outline the post-exposure prophylaxis for HIV infections (2004)

SN: HIV
SN: Pathogenesis of AIDS
LQ: Discuss the oportunistic infections in a case of AIDS (2002)
SN: AIDS
LQ: Classify the hepatitis viruses. Describe briefly about hepatitis C (2005)
SN: The slow viruses (2002)
SN: Rota virus (2001)
LQ: Write briefly on hepatitis B vaccine (2001)
SN: Icosahedral virus symmetry (2006)
Que: Enumerate arthropod-borne viruses commonly prevalent in India and describe laboratory diagnosis of any of them (2006)
SN: Strategies of HIV testing in India (2006)
Que: Describe briefly principle and uses of polymerase chain reaction (PCR) (2007)
SN: Inclusion bodies (2007)
Que: Describe briefly various methods of viral cultivation (2007)
Que: Discuss the laboratory markers associated with progession of HIV infection (2007)
Que: Describe the principle of ELISA. Enumerate the various types with one example each (2008)
Que: Discuss the opportunistic fungal infections of HIV/ AIDS (2008)
LQ: Enumerate 3 viruses transmitted by mosquito. Discuss the laboratory diagnosis of any one of these (2008)
LQ: Describe the principles and strategies for prevention and eradication of Poliomyelitis (2008).

E. MYCOLOGY AND MISCELLANEOUS

SN: Cryptococcus neoformans (2001)

SN: Cryptosporidiosis (2005)

SN: *Histoplasma capsulatum*

SN: Histoplasmosis

SN: Rhinosporidiosis (2005)

SN: Madura foot (1988)

SN: Write the technique and interpretation for testing antibiotic sensitivity by stroke's method

SN: *Candida albicans* (2002)

SN: Presumptive coliform count

LQ: Write briefly on *Candida albicans*. Enumerate opportunistic fungal infections in AIDS. (2004)

LQ: Enumerate the water-borne diseases and give laboratory diagnosis of any one of them

SN: Classify dermatophytes. Discuss the infection produced by them and their laboratory diagnosis

LQ: Define "Hospital acquired infections." Discuss the epidemiological markers used for its surveillance

LD: Hospital acquired infection

LQ: Write briefly on *Cryptococcus neoformans* (2001)

SN: Actinomycosis (2005)

LQ: Enumerate the various infections caused by Candida spp. Describe briefly the laboratory diagnosis of Candidiasis (2005)

LD: Superficial mycoses

SN: Dermatophytes

LQ: Write briefly about the universal precautions in health care setting (2002)

SN: Mycetoma (2002)

LQ: Define Biomedical waste. Discuss briefly its methods of disposal (2004)

LQ: Define hospital acquired infections. Discuss prevention and control of hospital acquired infections (2005)

SN: Presumptive coliform count (2006)

Que: Enumerate causes of mycetoma and discuss the laboratory diagnosis of any of the fingal causes (2006)

SN: Oral candidiasis (2006)

Que: Define biomedical waste. Discuss briefly its methods of disposal (2007)

Que: Name various genera of dermatophytes. Discuss the laboratory diagnosis of infections caused by dermatophytes. (2007)

SN: Rhinosporidiosis (2007)

Que: What are nosocomial infections? What is the role of a microbiologist in their control (2008)

SN: Cryptococcus neoformans (2008)

SN: Direct demonstration of fungi in clinical samples (2008).

F. PARASITOLOGY

LQ: Enumerate parasites found in blood. Describe the human life cycle of *P.vivax* (2005)

SN: Extraintestinal amoebiasis

SN: *Giardia lamblia* (2001)

LQ: Write a brief note on *Giardia lamblia* (2001)

SN: Cysticercus cellulosae (2004)

SN: Life cycle of *Echinococcus granulosum*

SN: Life cycle of *Plasmodium falciparum*

SN: Life cycle of *W. bancrofti*

SN: Pathogenesis and laboratory diagnosis of *Tenia solium*

SN: Pathogenic mechanism of diarrhoea by *E.coli*

SN: Pernicious malaria

SN: Primary amoebic meningoencephalitis

LQ: Describe briefly the morphology and life cycle of *Toxoplasma gondii* (2001)

LQ: Enumerate the parasites causing infection in AIDS patients. Outline the laboratory diagnosis of any one of them (2001)

SN: Hydatid cyst and laboratory diagnosis of the disease produced by it

SN: Life cycle of echinococcus granulosus and its pathogenicity

SN: Life cycle of pathogenicity of ankylostoma duodenale

LQ: Enumerate Plasmodia pathogenic to man. Discuss with the help of diagrams the life cycle of the parasite commonly associated with cerebral malaria and its laboratory diagnosis (2002)

LD: Extraintestinal amoebiasis.

LD: Hepatic amoebiasis.

SN: Free living amoeba (2002)

LD: Kala azar.

LQ: Enumerate tissue nematodes. Describe the life cycle of Guinea worm (2004)

LD: Malaria

LQ: Describe the life cycle and pathogenicity of entamoeba histolytica and the laboratory diagnosis of amoebiasis

SN: Post-kala-azar dermal Leishmaniasis (2005)

LQ: Describe the life cycle of *Wuchereria bancrofit*. Write briefly about occult filariasis.

LQ: Enumerate the haemoflagellates pathogenic for man and the diseases caused by them. Describe the laboratory diagnosis of any one of them

SN: Primary amoebic meningoencephalitis (2004)

LQ: Enumerate the tissue nematodes of man and give life cycle of any one of them

LQ: Enumerate the tissue nematodes. Describe the life cycle of *Dracunculus medinensis*

SN: Concentration method of stool examination (2000)

SN: Life cycle of *Dracunculus medinensis*

SN: Laboratory diagnosis fo kala-azar (2002)

Que: Describe briefly the morphology and life cycle of *Toxoplasma gondii* (2006)

SN: Cerebral malaria (2006)

SN: Life cycle of *Ascari lumbricoides* (2006)

Que: Describe the life-cycle of malarial parasite in details (2007)

SN: Amoebic liver abscess (2007)

SN: Casoni's test (2007).

Note:

LQ: Long Questions

SN: Short Note

LD: Laboratory Diagnosis

DW: Difference Between

Que: Question

Que: Describe the life cycle and diagnosis of the agent causing hydatid disease (2008)

SN: The differences between Plasmodium vivax and Plasmodium falciparum on peripheral blood smear examination (2008)

SN: Larva migrans (2008).

3. TOPICS FOR SPOTTING

⇨ Nutrient agar
⇨ Blood agar
⇨ Chocolate agar
⇨ Selenite F-broth
⇨ Wilson and Blair medium
⇨ McLeod's medium
⇨ Stuart's medium
⇨ Thayer-Martin medium
⇨ Pus culture swab
⇨ Nutrient broth
⇨ McIntosh Field's jar
⇨ ELISA kit
⇨ Blood culture bottle
⇨ Culture plate
⇨ Agar
⇨ Asbestos filters
⇨ Round worm
⇨ Stool slide for cysts/ova
⇨ Czapek-Dox medium
⇨ Postnatal swab (West's postnatal swab)
⇨ Ringworm
⇨ MacConkey's medium
⇨ Nagler's medium
⇨ Robertson's cooked medium
⇨ Durham's tube.

4. GRAM'S STAINING FOR PRACTICAL

Gram's stain = Devised by Christian gram in 1884
= Method of staining of bacteria in tissues.

Technique

Involves 4 steps (after fixing the slide).

Step 1: Primary staining with crystal voilet or methyl voilet or gentian voilet dye (60 sec).

Step 2: Application of dilute solution of iodine (60 sec).

Step 3: Discolouration with an organic solvent such as ethanol, acetone or aniline.

Step 4: Couterstaining with dye of contrast colour, e.g. carbol fuchin, safranine or neutral red (30 sec).

- Gram-positive bacteria
  = appear voilet = resist decolourization.
  = cells have more acidic protoplasm which may account for their retaining the basic primary dye.
- Gram-negative bacteria = appear red = decolourised by organic solvent and therefore take the counterstains.

Difference between cell walls of gram-positive and gram-negative bacteria

Gram-positive	Gram-negative
1. Thicker	1. Thinner
2. Few variety of amino acids	2. Several varieties of amino acids
3. Aromatic and sulphur containing amino acids are not present	3. Aromatic and sulphur containing amino acids are present
4. Lipids are absent or scanty	4. Lipids are present
5. Teichoic acid is present	5. Teichoic acid is absent

Few examples:

Gram-positive bacteria	Gram-negative bacteria
Staphylococcus aureus	*Neisseria gonorrhoea*
Staphylococcus albus	*Neisseria meningitidis*
Staph. citreus	Veillonella
Staph. pyogenes	Bacteroides
Staph epidermis	B. sphaerophonus
Streptococcus pyogenes	B. Dialister
Str. viridans	B. Fragilis
Str. faecalis	
Str. bovis	F. fusiformis
Str. equinus	Enterobacteriaceae
Str. pneumonia	Klebsiella
or *Diplococcus pneumonia*	Shigella sonnei
or *pneumococcus*	shigella
Corynebacterium diphtheriae	Salmonella
C. pseudotuberculosis	Escherichia
C. ulcerans	Citrobacter
Bacillus anthracis	Enterobacter
Clostridium welchii	Hafnia
Cl. tetani	*Vibrio cholerae*
	V. comma
Mycobacterium tuberculosis	Pseudomonas
	Yersinia pestis
M. leprae	*Haemophilus influenzae*

5. SPECIAL STRAINS FOR PRACTICALS (FOR ACID-FAST BACILLI)

Special stains important from practical point of view are following:
1. Zeihl-Neelsen staining.
2. Albert staining.

1. Zeihl-Neelsen Staining
⇨ Done for acid-fast bacilli, e.g. tubercle bacilli
⇨ Method
   • Fixing of slide (drying and fixing)
   • Application of strong solution of carbol fuschin and heating for 5 min
   • Washed with water
   • Decolourization with 20% H_2SO_4
   • Ninety five percent ethanol for 2 min
   • Counter staining with methylene blue for 1 min.
⇨ Acid-fast bacilli retain the red dye (fuschin)
⇨ Others take counterstain (methylene blue)
⇨ Acid fastness is due to high content and variety of lipids, fatty acids, in tubercle bacilli
⇨ Mycolic acid is also responsible for acid fastness
⇨ Acid fastness also depends on integrity of the cell wall
⇨ At least 10,000 acid-fast bacilli per ml should be present in sputum to be readily demonstrable in direct smears.
⇨ Grading of smear
   1 + = 3-9 bacilli in entire smear
   2 + = > 10 bacilli in smear
   3 + = > 10 bacilli seen in most oil immersion fields
⇨ Demonstration of acid-fast bacilli microscopically provides only presumptive evidence of tuberculosis as saprophytic mycobacteria also presents a similar appearance.
⇨ Other counter stains that can be used are:
   • 1% picric acid.
   • 0.2% malachito green.

2. Albert Staining Method
Stains used are Albert I and Albert II stain.

6. TOPICS FOR STOOL EXAMINATION

⇨ Occult blood
⇨ Cysts, ova, etc.
⇨ Entamoeba histolytica
⇨ Pus cells
⇨ Epithelial cells
⇨ Fresh blood.

7. TOPICS FOR THEORY VIVA

⇨ Microscope (types)
⇨ Staining of slide
⇨ Fixing of slide for staining
⇨ Bacterial growth curve
⇨ Sterilization of plastic material
⇨ Sterilization methods used in hospital
⇨ Autoclave
⇨ Testing of disinfectants
⇨ Simple media for culture
⇨ Indications of culture
⇨ Advantages of blood, urine, pus, semen culture
⇨ Selective media
⇨ MacConkey's medium
⇨ Thayer-Martin medium
⇨ Robertson's cooked meat media
⇨ Stuart's medium
⇨ Urine culture and sensitivity
⇨ Drug resistance
⇨ Infection
⇨ Various sources of infection
⇨ Control of infection
⇨ Diagnosis of infection
⇨ Exotoxins and endotoxins
⇨ Infectious diseases
⇨ Active and passive immunity
⇨ Local immunity
⇨ Antigen antibody reactions
⇨ Immunoglobulins
⇨ IgG, IgA, IgM
⇨ Immunoelectrophoresis
⇨ Radioimmunoassay
⇨ ELISA
⇨ Complement pathway
⇨ MHC (major compatibility complex)
⇨ Type I, II, III hypersensitivity
⇨ Tuberculosis—diagnosis and treatment
⇨ Infections caused by staphylococcus and streptococcus

⇨ Gonorrhoea and its treatment
⇨ Gas gangrene
⇨ *E. coli*
⇨ Intestinal pathogens
⇨ Body defence mechanisms
⇨ General properties of viruses
⇨ HIV (AIDS)
⇨ Universal precautions against AIDS
⇨ Hospital acquired infections
⇨ Common fungal infections—diagnosis and treatment
⇨ Fungal culture.

8. LABORATORY DIAGNOSIS OF SOME COMMON INFECTIONS

A. LABORATORY DIAGNOSIS OF SORE THROAT

1. Organisms associated with acute sore throat:

Bacterial	Viral	Fungal
Strep. pyogenes group A	Rhinovirus	Candida albicans
C. diphtheria	Coronavirus	
Staph. aureus (MRSA)	Adrenovirus	
H. influenzae	Parainfluenza	
Borrelia vincents	Coxsackie	Others
N. gonorrhea	EBV	
Strep pyogenes group C, D	Herpes simplex 1,2	Agranulocytosis
		Acute leukemia

Sample Collection

1. Throat swab
   - 2 samples, cotton swab is used)
   - Dacron/Ca—aliginate swabs better (cotton has acids which are inhibitory to certain organisms).
2. Nasopharyngeal swabs: esp for Neisseria, Borrelia.

Transport

- Immediately otherwise refrigeration.
- Stuart's/Pike's transport media.

Microscopy

1. Gram's stain (Strep, *C. diphtheria*, Staph., Candida., Borrelia)
2. Albert's stain: for *C. diphtheria*
3. Fat for detection of antigen esp. in viral infections
   Kits for Inf: Parainfl., *S. pyogenes*, *H. influenzae* are available.

Culture

1. Blood agar: Staph., Strep., *C. diphtheria*, Candida (opaque pasty).
2. LSS: for *C. diphtheria*
3. KTBA: for *C. diphtheria*
4. Crystal violet blood agar: for *Strep pyogenes.*
5. Saboraud's dextrose agar: for Candida.
6. Tissue culture for viruses: look for CPE.

Identification

I. Strep
   1. Biochem
      a. Catalase -ve
      b. PYR hydrolysis +ve.
   2. Bacitracin sensitivity +ve for *Strep. pyogenes.*
   3. Lancefield's grouping.
II. *C. diphtheriae*
   1. Albert's straining–metachromatic granules, cuneiform.
   2. Biochemi: Glu, maltose, mannose (acid only).
   3. Immunofluorescence.
   4. Toxigenicity testing.
III. Vincent's angina
    Gram's stain:
    • Fusospirotrichosis
    • Stender borelia can be seen with large, spindle shaped gram -ve fusobacteria.
IV. Candida
   1. Growth on blood agar.
   2. Chlamydospores formation on corn meal agar culture at 20° C.
   3. Raynaud's Braude phenomenon, i.e. formation of germ tubes within 24 hrs in human serum at 37° C.
V. Viruses
   1. CPE in tissue cultures.
   2. Immunology.
   3. For infectious mononucleosis: Paul Bunnel test.

B. LABORATORY DIAGNOSIS OF DIPHTHERIA

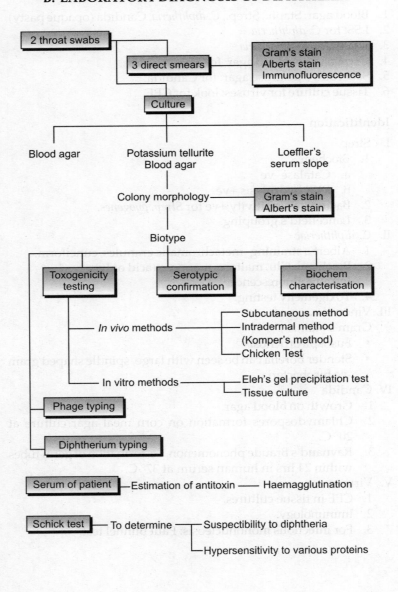

Sample

1. Throat swab
   - Done in good light using tongue depressor
   - Begin in the site of maximum inflammation, rub it viorously, pull out a portion of pseudomembrane.
2. Serum.
3. Scrapings from lesions.

Transport

If delay in innoculation keep it moistened in sterile horse serum.

Direct Smear

1. *Gram's stain:* Gram +ve, club shaped, cuneiform arrangement.
2. *Albert's stain:* Metachromatic granules, cuneiform arrangement.
3. *Immunofluorescence:* Rapid and sensitive method.

Culture

1. LSS: 75 percent serum in glucose broth. Make solid by inspissation
   Advantages:
   - Only 6-8 hrs required for growth
   - ↑ metachromatic granules
   - Biochemical tests from growth
   - Animal pathogenicity from growth
2. Blood agar:
   - In 24 hrs gray glistening colonies
   - To rule out other organisms (Staph/Strep pharyngitis)
3. KTBA: (0.04% potassium tellurite)
   Imp. For isolation from carriers, contacts and convalescents.
   In 48 hrs—Black coloured colonies.

   Daisy head   Frog's egg   Poached egg

Identification

1. Smear from culture
   Gram's staining
   Albert's staining.

2. Biochemical tests
   a. Hiss's serum sugars
      Glucose, maltose +ve (acid only), Sucrose -ve
   b. Urease -ve
   c. Phosphatase +ve.
3. Serotyping confirmatory.

Toxigenicity Tests

1. *In vivo*   Subcutaneous method
              Intradermal method.
2. *In vitro* Elck's gel precipitation test
              Tissue culture.

Others

Typing   Phage typing
          Diphtheriocin typing.

Serology

Estimation of antitoxin by haemagglutination.

Schick's Test

To determine
a. Susceptibility to diphtheria.
b. Hypersensitivity to various proteins.

Differential Diagnosis

1. *Strep. pyogenes:* White pustular spot on tonsil and post-pharyngeal wall.
2. Vincent's angina.   ⎤ White gray membranous
3. Oral thrush due to *Candida*   ⎬ patch
   albicans.   ⎦
4. Diphtheria.
5. *Staph. pharyngitis*.

C. LABORATORY DIAGNOSIS OF MENINGITIS

1. Organisms Causing Meningitis

Pyogenic meningitis	Aseptic meningitis	Chronic meningitis
Strep pneumoniae	Cryptococcus neoformans	Mycobacterium tuberculosis
Pneumococcus	Naegleria	Cryptococcus neoformans
H. influenzae	Acanthamoeba	Histoplasma capsulatum
N. meningitidis	Candida	Candida
Strep agalactiae	Viruse: Polio,	
Streptococcus	Coxsackie A and B	Taenia solium
Group B	Mumps, measles,	Entamoeba histolytica
Listeria	Herpes simplex	
monocytogenes	Herpes zoster	
Staphylococcus		

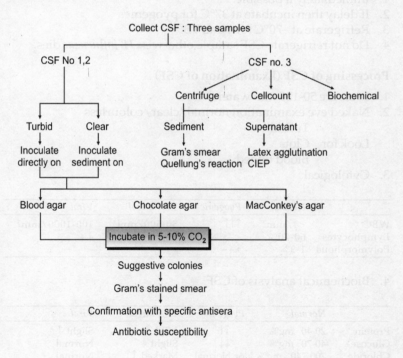

Collect CSF : Three samples

CSF No 1,2   CSF no. 3

CSF no. 3 → Centrifuge, Cellcount, Biochemical

Turbid — Inoculate directly on

Clear — Inoculate sediment on

Centrifuge → Sediment — Gram's smear / Quellung's reaction

Centrifuge → Supernatant — Latex agglutination / CIEP

Blood agar   Chocolate agar   MacConkey's agar

Incubate in 5-10% CO_2

Suggestive colonies

Gram's stained smear

Confirmation with specific antisera

Antibiotic susceptibility

Samples

1. CSF: 3-5 by Lumbar puncture in Bijou bottles
   a. Plain bottle
   b. 2 cc, Glucose broth.
2. Blood: For culture serology. Incubate for 4-7 days with daily subcultures.
3. Nasopharyngeal swab:
   West's postnatal swab for carriers
   Kept in Stuart's medium.
4. Petechial skin lesions: M/E and cultur .
5. Throat washings and faeces: for viral.

Transport

1. Immediately if possible.
2. If delay then incubate at 37°C for pyogenic.
3. Refrigerate at –70°C for viral, TB.
4. Do not refrigerate CSF sample otherwise *H. influenzae* dies.

Processing of CSF (Examination of CSF)

1. Pressure 50-180 mm water.
2. Naked eye examination normal/clear/colourless
   Turbidity
   Look for   Clots
             Blood tinged.
3. Cytological.

	Normal	Pyogenic	TB/Fungal	Viral
WBC	<4/mm³	↑↑↑	50-500/mm³	100-1000/mm³
Lymphocytes	60-70%	-	++	++
Polymorphous	1-3%	+++	-	-

4. Biochemical analysis of CSF

	Normal	Pyogenic	TB/Fungal	Viral
Protein	20-40 mg%	↑↑	Mild ↑	Slight ↑
Glucose	40-70 mg%	↓↓	Slight ↓	Normal
Chloride	700-740 mg% ↓ or Normal		Marked ↑↑	Normal

5. Smear:
   A. Wet film
      1. Cell counting slide/plain slide.
      2. No of pus cells/PMN.
      3. Can also detect free living amoeba and yeast.
   B. Gram staining
      1. Gram +ve/Gram -ve.
      2. Morphology (meningitidis, pneumoniae, *H. influenzae*).
   C. India ink: For cryptococcus and pneumococcus (capsulated organisms).
   D. ZN staining: If TB suspected.
   E. Acridine orange fluoroschrome staining
      1. Rapid and sensitive.
      2. All bacteria stained by it.
6. Serology: Use supernatant
   1. Latex agglutination, CIEP, IF.
   2. *Staph. aureus* coagglutination.
   3. Limulus lysin test (LPS is gram -ve).
   4. Neurosyphilis: VDRL, TPHA.
   5. IgG, IgA, IgM index.
   6. Reverse Western Blot Assay (for TB).
7. Culture
   1. Blood agar.
   2. MacConkey agar.
   3. Chocolate agar.
   4. CSF ⟨ with Glucose broth
         without Glucose broth.
   5. For *H. influenzae* Filde's agar
      TB LJ medium.
   6. Viral: Inoculate into appropriate cell culture directly.

Identification

1. Neisseria
   a. Colony—1 mm, round, convex, translucent, smooth, glistening, lenticular shape, easily emulsifiable, butyrous consistency.

b. Biochem: Catalase +ve, Oxidase +ve (prompt oxidase and Kovae's method).

c. Serology: Agglutination with specific antisera.

2. Pneumococcus

a. Colony: 0.5-1 mm, dome-shaped, round, glistening

b. Biochem: Quellung's +ve, insulin fermentation, bile soluble, optochin sensitivity.

c. Serology: Precipitation of SSb with specific antisera.

3. *H. influenzae*

a. Indescence on Filde's agar.

b. Quellung's with Type B antisera.

c. Capsular polysaccharide Ppt with antisera.

Antibiotic Sensitivity

With penicillin, Chloramphenicol, Streptomycin.

D. LABORATORY DIAGNOSIS OF DIARRHEA

Common Causes of GI Illness

1. Bacteria
     Vibrio cholerae 0137, EI Tor
     E.coli (ETEC, EIEC, EPEC, EHEC)
     Salmonella spp, except *S. typhi*/paratyphi
     Campylobacter species
     γ parahemolyticus
     Yersinia enterocolitica
     Plesiomonas
     Shigelloides
     Aeromonas
     S. typhimunum: Septicaemia in rats, mild diarrhea in humans.
2. Protozoa
     Entamoeba histolytica
     Giardia lamblia
     Cryptosporidium parvum opportunistic
     Balantidum coli: flagellae.
3. Helminth
     Cystosomenas
     Brunchumella.
4. Viruses
     Rotavirus mainly in paediatric are group, coronavirus, Norwalk virus
     Astrovirus
     Calcivirus
     SRS virus (Small rounded structural viruses)
     Adenovirus.
5 Fungus
     Candida albicans ——Children
     ＼Older immunocompromised.
6. Antibiotic associated colitis
     Clostridium difficile
     Staph. enterocolitis
     Candida.

Food Poisoning: Causative Agents

I. Infective
   A. Nontoxin mediated
      - Salmonella species
      - Campylobacter species
      - Vibrio parahemolyticus
      - Bacillus aureus.
   B. Toxin mediated
      - *Staphylococcus aureus*
      - *Clostridium perfringens*
      - *Clostridium botulinum*
      - *E. coli* (toxin producing) (0157 H7 vertotoxin).
II. Noninfective
   A. Allergic
      - Shell fish
      - Strawberries.
   B. Nonallergic
      - Fish
      - Mushrooms
      - Chemicals, etc.

Specimen Collection

- Appropriate stool in a wide mouth bottle
- Well collected containing mucus and stool
- Correctly labelled.

Transport

Rapid and safe, reach the lab in 1 hour.

Reception

Match slip and sample
Record
Assign lab number.

Cultivation/Isolation

Preliminary identity (day 1 after receipt)——— Biological
                                          Biochemical

Identification AST

Final report (2nd day).

Further

Typing
Toxin production   } Supplementary report
Antibiotic sensitivity test

Collection and Transport of Stool Specimen

- Clean, wash cardboard or plastic container
- Reach lab within one hour
- Avoid preservatives, quantity 1 tsp (about 5 ml)
- If delay exported use transport medium
    Cary Blair medium: Yersinia
    Buffered glycerol saline
- Stool for virus detection
- Use of Stuart's Transport medium
- Rectal swabs
- Additional specimens.

Culture of Bacteriological Agents

1. Blood agar (Trypticase Soy agar + 5% sheep blood).
2. MacConkey agar   Selective bacteria
                       Late lactose fermenter: *S. sonni*
   XLD.
3. Highly selective: Brilliant green Bismuth sulphite medium
       S. typhi → Black
       Others → Pink
   35-37°C for   24-48 hrs
   for 0157 H7 verotoxin *E. coli*
       Sorbitol MacConkey (1% sorbitol in place of lactose)
       Unable to ferment (15% *E. coli* do)
       Detect toxin by cell culture assay.

Enrichment Medium

Liquid medium which support growth
    Selenite F broth
    Tetrathionate broth

Campylobacter → Blood agar: *C. jejuni, coli*
  42°C for 24-48 hrs
H. pylori →   Urease test
         Urease smell test
TCBS → Vibrio
CIN medium agar → Yersinia enterocolitica
Crystal violet, Neural red, Mannitol +.

Others

Toxin assay, phate typing, antibiogram.

E. LABORATORY DIAGNOSIS OF GAS GANGRENE

Specimen

1. Film's flora
   a. Affected tissue
   b. Necrotic tissue
   c. Wound exudate.
2. Exudate from depth of wound by pipette or swab.
3. Necrotic tissue and muscle fragments.

Transport

1. Stuart's medium.
2. RCM.
3. Thioglycollate broth.
4. PRAS (per reduced anaerobic sterilized) medium.

Direct Smear

1. *Gram's stain:* To identity the species and their relative number.
   Boxcar appearance: rods stout, thick, spores are colourless
   Cl. welchii → large no; regularly shaped, gram +ve, bacilli without spores.
   Cl. speticum → Citron bodies and boat or leaf shaped, pleomorphic bacilli, irregular staining.
   Cl. edematiene → large bacilli with oval subterminal spores.
   Cl. tetani → slender bacilli, round terminal spores.

Culture

Both aerobic and anaerobic cultures done.
1. RCM 4 tubes of RCM broth are inoculated and heated at 100°C for 5, 10, 15, 20 minutes. Incubate and subculture on blood agar 24-48 hours to differentiate organisms with heat resistant spore.
2. Fresh Horse Blood agar ⎤ • All contain egg yolk hence
3. Blood agar with neomycin ⎟ can be used for Naegler's
4. Heated blood agar ⎟ reaction
5. Lowburry's and Lilly's ⎦ • 5-6% agar used to prevent
   medium swarming.
6. Brain heart infusion agar → better than BA (used in MAMC).
   After 1-2 days of incubation on above media look for wine-leaf colonies.

Motility (in anaerobes)

1. Wet smear with cover slip preparation sealed with nail enamel.
2. Capillary tube method seal both ends and look in phase contrast micro or light micro.
3. Stab innoculation of semisolid agar: paraffin on top. Incubate, if mobile, growth away from central stab line (feathering effect).

Identification

1. Naegler's reaction.
2. Stormy fermentation.
3. Gas liquid chromatography: detect production of butyric acid.
4. Animal pathogenicity filtrate of RCM in thigh of guinea pig → necrosis → death Coastrol animal with antitoxin → no death.

F. HOSPITAL ACQUIRED INFECTIONS

Definition

Any clinical reconcilable and microbiological disease which affect the patients as because of his getting admitted to hospital or just visit or to work in the hospital staff or effect of:
1. History
2. The host triad
3. Type of HAI
4. Investigation
5. Control.
1. Environment

   Living personelle → infect other patient

   Non-living: room, solution, instrument, air, water.
2. Source of infection: Temporary origin of infection (site of bacteria for short period)

   Reservoir → permanent site (not multiply) chemical

   Env → Dry, gram +ve infection—cocci—staph (not strep.)
   - → Wet gram -ve rods

     Enterobacteria: *E. coli*, Kleb

     Non-enterobacteriacea: Pseudomonas, Helicobacter (grow in savalon, dettol).
   - → Direct contaminated food, surface, air, surface (Air: tiny particles, long disease, e.g. TB)

     Droplet nucleus.
   - → Indirect source—organisms (human and non-human vehicle)

   Vector borne and material borne (esp in newborn).
3. Factors → the risk of HAI

Patient	Procedure/Hospital
• Age	• Prolonged stay
• Sex	• ICU case
• Underlying disease	• Invasive procedure
• Immunocompromise	• Intubation
• Loss of skin	
• Obesity	
• Malnutrition	

Apache Score

Agent: Organisms: True trends of pathogens involved in HAI
1. Urinary tract infection: *E. coli*, serrata, klebsiella.
2. Surgical site: Gram +ve (staph).

3. Resp site: Gram -ve rods, Strep., Pneumoniae, *Kleb Pneum., Staph aureus.*
4. Bloodstream: Gram +ve cocci—major cause of death before strep.

Agent (Organisms)

1. *Strep pyogenes*—in neonates from nurse → but high mortality.
2. *Staph. aureus*—MRSA, SMRSA.
3. CNS (catalase negative staphylococcus).
4. *S. typhi.*
5. Salmonella spp.
6. Shigella.
7. *Cl. perfringens.*
8. Enterobacteriacea.
   (Kleb, *E. coli*, Proteus, Providencia, Enterobacter, Serratia).
9. *Pseudomonas*, aeruginosa spp.
10. Legionella.
11. HIV and hepatitis B.

Source

- Estrogenous living person—cross infection
  Non-living—environmental infection
- Endogenous: from patient himself—resistant development.

Site (Most common)

- UTI continuous and difficult in Rx
  - Thirty three percent in all, gram -ve rods > gm +ve cocci > candida
  - In young and now CNS on the head
  - UTI common if female, underlying usual disease, exterile age, catheterization, diarrhea.
- Surgical site injection: 15 percent, usually present after discharge from hospital.
  - - gm + ve cocci + gm -ve rods > candida
  - site injection: 15 percent, usually present after discharge from hospital
  - - gm + ve cocci + gm -ve rods > candida
  - Common if age, female preoperative sharing, obesity, DM, malnutrition, duration of surgery, preoperative stay
    Wound Clean
       Clean contaminated
       Contaminated.

- RTI: 15-16%
  - Increased mortality
  - Usually pneumonia
  - GNR > gP > Pneumonia
  - Factors: Long duration
      Comatose patient
      Ventilatory support
      Antacid Rx.
- Bloodstream infection
  - 15%: ↑↑ mortality

Incidence

Endemic: 5-10 percent is expected within hospital.
Epidemic: 20-30 percent → normal, our hospital: 44 percent.
Hospital outbreak: caused—unusual pathogen: salmonella
    Virulent pathogen
    Highly multidrug resistant esp. Pseudomonas.

High-risk Area

1. ICU
2. Nurseries
3. Postoperative ward
4. Burns ward
5. Haemodialysis unit
6. Cancer wards
7. HIV wards
8. Geriatric wards
9. Transplant unit

Outbreak Pathogen

1. *Strep. pyogenes*
2. EMRSA
3. VRE
4. *Clostridium perfringens,* difficile
5. Resistant gram-negative: Acromonas, Enterobacter, Pseudomonas, others
6. Salmonella—STM
7. WTD
8. Pneumococcal

9. Legionella
10. Mycobacteria.

Laboratory Diagnosis

1. Epidemiological: Hypothesis likely source and reservoir.
2. Mycobacterial: Prove the source
   1. Identification of pathogen (depends upon site involved)
      - Collection of sample
      - Transport
      - Culture enrichment media—solid/liquid
      - Biochemical
      - AB sensitivity.
   2. Typing most important in diagnosis.
      - Method with subdivide gp otherwise identical belong to same spectes by single character.
      - Classified: Phenotyping—conventional method. Genotyping—molecular.

Phenotyping

1. Morpho typing → colony morphology.
2. Serotyping: antigenic, O, H, K.
3. Biotyping—biochemical.
4. Bacteriocin typing → sensitivity/resistant to std bact.
5. Phage → phage susceptibility (e.g. *S. typhi*, Staph).
6. Antibiogram.
7. Resistogram—to heavy metab.
8. Auxotype: Auxotrope (Bact) undergoes.
9. Protein profile: Electrophoresis
                       Outer membrane protein.

Genotyping

1. Chromosomal material
2. Plasmid drug
   - Small and easily extract
   - Disadvantage not present in all bacteria
   - DNA → broken y endonucleases → banding pattern

3. Other methods
   - Southern blotting
   - Ribotyping
   - PCR.

Sampling should also be done to find the source of infection:
   a. Surface sampling
   b. Staph sampling: nasal swab, perineal swab, hand swab
   Typing should be done.

Control

Medical superintendent → Infection control committee → team.

G. LABORATORY DIAGNOSIS OF UTI

Upper UTI

- Renal pelvis and ureter
- Pain radiates down
- Fever with chills and agar
- Associated with DM and pregnancy
- All age groups
- Same for both sexes
- Infection males—prostate catheterisation.

Lower UTI

- Urinary bladder and urethra
- Cystitis dysuria
- Pass urine at small intervals
- More common in (shorter urethra, proximity of urethra to anus)
- Change in genitourinary tract in menopausal age
- First trimester of pregnancy
- Contraceptive foam gels.

Precipitating Factors

- Diabetes
- Neurogenic disorder
- Retention due to obstruction
  Parts surrounding areas have commensals. Coliforms get entry from surrounding to urethra.

Ascending from urethra: Cystitis, enterobacterium.

Descending from blood: Mycobacterium, Salmonella.

Causes

1. Gram -ve: *E. coli,* Proteus, Pseudomonas, Klebsiella, Citrobacter, Salmonella, Edwardsiella
2. Gram +ve: Staphylococcus
   Aureus
   Epidermis (catheterisation)
   Saprophyticus.
3. Candida.

4. Strep⎯B
        ⎯D.
5. Viruses: CMV, Adenovirus.
6. Parasites: Trichomonas vaginalis, Schistosomia hematobium.

Sample Collection

Urine • Midstream: Clean catch tech
     • Suprapubic
     • Catheter sample.

Than catch: Preferred to be collected in the morning collect in sterile container urethral area is to be cleaned with soap.
   Midstream sample collected and timed send to lab
   Ideally two specimens collected.

Suprapubic specimen: Under aseptic conditions suprapubic puncture is done and urine is taken out.

Other Specimens Collected after Cystoscopy

Ab coated Bacteria test (for kidney)
   Urine is centrifuged
   Deposits have bacteria with fl. tagged antihemoglobulin
   Seen under UV light
   1/4 tbs bacteria emit fl. → infection in kidney.
Anaerobic culture of urine—never done
   Done from nephrostomy tube or Suprapubic catheter.

Transport

   Transport immediately
   Ideally processed within an hour
   If delayed keep in refrigerator 4°C for max 24 hours put certain chemicals glycerol/boric acid in container and urine is passed (stabilisers).

Wet Coverslip Preparation

   Directly made for   RBCs
                Casts
                Pus cells
                Crystals
                Bacteria

> 10 Pus cells/HPF → infection.

Uncentrifuged sample > 10 polymorplis → Infection

Gram's stain with one drop of urine

1 bac/field in 20 fields → infection.

Quantitative Culture

1. **Caliberated loop technique:** Counted according to mass diam of loop is standardised loop is put in the container and taken out straight (quantity - 0.01 ml.)

   Put in culture plate centre. Put line upwards and downwards and in a zig zag manner.

Incubate 24 hrs × 37°C — colony count

100,000 bacteria/ml—contamination

In patient on antimicrobial therapy or org. line *Staph aureus* low count is important.

2. Pour Plate Method

Dilution of urine 1:10, 1:100 1:1000 in distilled H_2O in sterile petridish then put on nutrient agar media

Incubate overnight. After counting × by dilution factor growth on MacConkey.

E.coli	vs	Klebsiella
• Bright pink		• Large mucoid colonies of varying degrees of stick.

- Growth of proteus on blood agar
    Put refactive odour, fisley or seminal
    Swarming—striking feature of Pr vulgaris and mirabilis
    Det by motility.
- Growth of pseudomonas on nutrient agar
    Iridescent patches with a metallic sheet.

- Growth of *Staph. auerus* of on blood agar
  Large circular convex smooth shiny opaque easily emulsifiable
  Most strains are hemolytic (20-25% CO_2)
- Candida questained smear
  Budding gram +ve cells.

Chemical Methods

Not sensitive (used for presumptive of significant bacteria).
1. Griess nitrate test: Urine nitrite is absent (due to nitrate reducing bacteria).
2. Catalase test: Bacteremia hematuria.
3. TTC test: PPT of pink red colour in reagent caused by respiratory activity of growing bacteria.
4. Glucose test paper.
5. Dip slide culture: Agar coated slides are immersed in urine or even exposed to the stream of urine during voiding, incubated and growth estimated by colony count or by color change of indicators (Most sensitive and reliable test).

Automated Techniques

1. Bacitracin.
2. Unscreen.

Antibiotic Sensitivity Testing

Amikacin
Gentamicin
Norfloxacin
Nalidixic acid
Netlimycin.

9. IMPORTANT POINTS

⇨ **SOME USEFUL STAINS**

1. Iron	⇨	Pearls (Prussian blue)
	⇨	KF_3CN, HCl
	⇨	FFl → Blue.
2. Calcium	⇨	Von Kossen.
3. Amyloid	⇨	Methyl violet
	⇨	Congo red
	⇨	Thioflavin.
4. Fat	⇨	Oil red O
	⇨	Sudan black B
5. Glycogen	⇨	PAS.
6. LFD (liver)	⇨	PAS with diastase.
7. Staining for reticulocyte		
Supravital	⇨	New methylene blue
	⇨	Brilliant crystalline blue.

⇨ **Q FEVER**

Coxiella Burneti (in urine) among rickettsias is usually transmitted to human and not by arthropods but by inhalation or ingestion.

Transmission

By cows and goats is principally through feces, placenta and milk inhalation of contaminated dust and of droplets from infected animal tissue is main source of human infection. There is no man to man transmission.

Clinical Findings

Symptoms and Signs

After incubation period of 1-3 weeks febrile illness develop with headache.

Nonproductive cough

Acute phase → granulomatous, hepatitis

Chronic (rare) endocarditis, encephalitis, hemolytic anemia, orchitis.

Laboratory findings

- ↑ LFT, leucocytosis
- ↓ complement fixing.

D/D

Viral, mycoplasma, bact. pneumonia, brucellosis, TB.

Prevention

Detection of injection in live stock reduction of contact with infected animal or dust contaminated clotes.

A vaccine of formalin inactivated phase I coxelia is being developed for high risk cases.

Treatment

- Tetracycline (25 mg/kg/day)
- Doxycycline (100 mg BD).

➡ **Pasteurisation of Milk**

1. Holder's method = 63°C for 30 min
2. Flash process = HTST method = 72°C for 15-20 sec.
3. UHT method = 125°C for few seconds and then rapid cooling.

➡ **Types of filters**

1. Candle filters
   a. Unglazed ceramic filters= chamberland and Doulton filters
   b. Diatomaceous earth filters = Bankerfeld and Mendler filders
2. Asbestos filters = Seitz and Sterimant filters
3. Sintered glass filters
4. Membrane filters = APD = 0.22 µm (average)

➡ **Interleukins**

IL-1 and IL -8 are produced by macrophages
IL-7, IL-11 are produced by marrow stromal cells and all others are produced By T cells.

➡ Combined immunization = Active + passive immunization.
➡ The most common cause of severe combined immunodeficiency disease (SCID) is the deficiency of enzyme ADA (Adenosine deaminase).

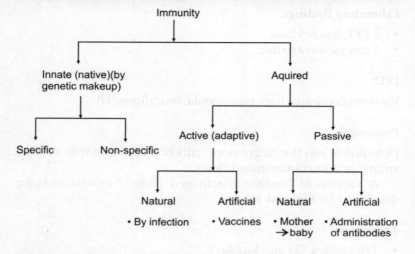

⇨ IgG = Normally transported across placeta, MC IgG = IgG_1

⇨ IgM= Earliest immunoglobulin synthesized by the fetus and its presence in fetus or newborn indicates intrauterine infection.
  – Detection in serum indicates recent infection
  – Mediates primary immune response.

⇨ IgE = Mostly extravascular, shortest ½ life and is responsible for anaphylactic type hypersensitivity.

⇨ Antigens are classified as T- cell dependent (TD) and T-cell independent (TI).

⇨ Antibody production is the property of B cells.

⇨ Passively administered IgG suppresses the homologus antibody production by a "Feedback Mechanism" in isoimmunization of women by anti-Rh(D) Ig during/after delivery.

⇨ Lymphoid organs:

A. Central ⟨ Thymus = T cells = cellular immunity (CMI)

Bone marrow = B cells= Humoral immunity.

B. Peripheral
  1. Lymph nodes
  2. Spleen
  3. Mucosa associated lymphoid tissue (MALT)

⇨ Macrophages
- in blood = monocytes
- in tissue = Histiocytes

⇨ Microphages = Basophils, neutrophils, eosinophils.

⇨ Serological antigen antibody reactions:

1. Precipitation reactions

   Applications

   a. Ring test

   b. Slide test = (VDRL for syphilis) slide flocculation

   c. Tube test = (Kahn test for syphilis) Tube flocculation

   d. Immunodiffusion
   - Single/double diffusion in one direction
   - Single/double diffusion in two diffusions.
   - Immunoelectrophoresis

   e. Electroimmuno diffusion.

2. Agglutination reactions

   Application:

   a. Slide Agglutination = (BGCM) → (BG, CM)

   b. Tube Agglutination = (Widal test, Weil-Fleix test, Paul Bunnel test)

   Typhus fever
   Infectious mononucleosis

   c. Antiglobulin test = Coomb's test = direct/indirect

   d. Passive agglutination – (Rose-Waller test) – Rheumatoid arthritis
   - Latex agglutination test = for detection of CRP, ASO, RA factor, HCG etc.

⇨ The reaction between antigen and antibody occur in 3 stages.

   1. Primary stage

   2. Secondary stage = precipitation, agglutination, nevtralization of toxins, etc.

   3. Tertiary stage= clinical allergy, humoral immunity against infection diseases

⇨ Host versus graft response = Graft rejection.

⇨ Graft versus host response (GVH) reaction) = Graft mounts an immune response against the antigens of the host.

⇨ **Hypersensitivity:**

Type 1 = IgE type = Anaphylaxis
- Local eczema, Hay fever, asthma (atopy)
- Systemic: anaphylaxis

Examples: Theobald Smith's phenomenon, PK Reaction, Casoni's test

Type 2 = Cytotoxic = Antibody mediated damage, complement mediated, phagocytosis (IgGM) change in cellular function.

Examples = Blood transfusion reactions, hemolytic anaemia, Thrombocytopenia Grave's disease, *M. gravis*, ITP, Good Pasture's syndrome.

Type 3 = Immune complex phenomenon (IgM and IgG)
- Local: arthrus reaction
- Systemic: serum sickness

Examples: Schick's test, Post-streptococcal GN.

Type 4 = Delayed hypersensitivity : cellular immunity

Examples: Tuberculin test, Lepromin test, contact dermatitis, chronic graft rejection

⇨ All classes of Ig do not fix complement only IgM, TgG 3,1,2 fix complement (in this order)

⇨ Biological effects of C
1. Mediates immunological membrane damage
2. Amplify the inflammatory response
3. Antiviral activity
4. Interacts with coagulation
5. Bacteriolysis and cytolysis
6. Facilitates the uptake and destruction of pathogen by phagoaftic cells.
7. Participates in type II, III hypersensitivity reactions.

⇨ Complements are synthesized in intestinal epithelium (C_1), Macrophages (C_2, C_4) Spleen (C_5, C_8) and liver (C_3, C_6, C_9).

⇨ The HLA complex of genes is located on short arms of chromosome 6.

⇨ HLA and disease association:
1. HLA B27 =
   - Arthritis
     - Psoriatic arthritis
     - Reactive arthritis
     - Juvenile rheumatoid arthritis
   - Ankylosing spondylitis
   - Reiter's disease
2. HLA B-8 = Myasthenia gravis and hyperthyroidism (Grave's)
3. HLA DWa/DR_4 = Rheumatoid arthritis.
4. HLA DR_3 =
   - Myasthenia gravis (with B8)
   - Coelic disease (Gluten sensitive enteropathy)
   - Diabetes mellitus type 1 (Also DR_2, DR_4)

⇨ Types of graft
1. Autograft = to self (homograft to the same sexes)
2. Isograft = Different individual, genetically identical (Indentical twin)
3. Allograft = Genetically unrelated individual of same species.
4. Xenograft = Different species.

⇨ Transmission of genetic material (In bacteria)
1. Transformation = through the agency of free DNA
2. Transduction = through bacteriophage (virus)
3. Conjugation = through physical contact

⇨ Lysozymes are present in all body secretions and fluids except CSF, urine and sweat.

⇨ Memory T cells can be indentified by = 45 RD marker
Subset T cells (Medullary thymocytes) = 45 RA marker
All leukocytes = 45 RB marker
Subset T cells (medullary thymocytes) = 45 RC marker

⇨ Systemic classification of fungi:
1. Phycomycetes = Lower fungi
2. Ascomycetes = form sexual spores (ascospores)
3. Basidiomycetes = from sexual and pores (basidiospored) on a base
4. Fungi imperfecti = sexual phase have not been identified.

⇨ Skin test with Histoplasmosis demonstrates histoplasmosis (intracellular infection of reticuloendothelial system caused by histoplasma capsulatum).

⇨ Dermatophytes:
1. Trichophyton infects = Skin, hair, nails
2. Microsponim infects = Skins, hair
3. Epidermophytin infects = Skin, nails

DOC is Griseofulvin oral (duration of treatment) is Griseofulvin
- Skin = 3 wks
- Palm and soles = 4-6 wks
- Finger nails = 4-6 months
- Toe nails = 8-12 months

⇨ Dimorphic fungi
Blastomycete
Histoplasmosis   ⎤
Coccidioidomycosis ⎦ = Systemic infection
Sporotrichosis   = Subcutaneous infection

⇨ Prophylaxis against rabies in humans:
1. Active immunization (cell culture vaccines)
   a. Pre-exposure = 0, 7, 21 OR 0, 28, 56 days (3 doses)
   b. Post-exposure = 0,3,7,14, 30 and 90 days (optional) (5 doses)
2. Passive immunization
   HRIG = Human rabies immuneglobulin = dose = 20 IU/kg body weight of HRIG

⇨ Prophylaxis in animals: (Cell culture vaccines containing in activated viruses)
   Single IV injection at 12 wk of age and repeated 1-3 years interval

⇨ Vaccines for rabies:
1. Neural vaccines
   • Sample vaccine
   • BPL vaccine
   • Infant brain vaccine
2. Non-neural vaccines
   • Egg vaccines
   • Tissue/cell culture vaccines
   • Subunit vaccines

⇨ Schedule for neural vaccine

Class of patient	Sample vaccines	BPL vaccine
Class I	2 ml × 7 days	2 ml × 7 days
Class II	5 ml × 14 days	3 ml × 10 days
Class III	10 ml × 14 days	5 ml × 10 days

⇨ Classification of exposure (rabies)
Class I : Slight risk
   • Licks on healthy unbroken skins
   • Consumption of unboiled milk of suspected animal
   • Scratches without oozing blood

Class II : Moderate risk
   • Licker on fresh cuts
   • Secretches with oozing blood
   • All bites except those on head, neck, face palm and finger
   • Minor wounds < 5 in number

Class III: Severe risk
   • All bites with oozing blood on head, neck, fair, palm and finger
   • Lacerated wound on any part of the body
   • Multiple wounds > 5 in number
   • Bikes from wild animals.

⇨ Borrelia burgdorferi = Lyme's disease
⇨ B. Vincenti = Vincenti's angina
⇨ B. Recurrentis = relapsing fever
⇨ Cidex = 2% Gluteraldehyde solution.
⇨ Lapra cells = Histiocytes/macrophages
⇨ Generation time
  Coliform bacilli = 20 min
  Tubercle bacilli = 20 hrs
  Lapra bacilli = 20 days
⇨ Syphilis = Earliest test = FTA-ABS = most sensitive
  = most specific = TPI
⇨ Culture media for chlamydia = Mc Coy cell culture
⇨ Typhoid (diagnosis clue) ulcers = longitudinal (Transverse in TB)
  B = Blood culture is possive in 1 wk
  A = Antibodies (widal) in 2nd wk = maximum in 3rd wk
  S = Stool culture in max in 3rd wk
  U = Urine culture in max in 4th wk
⇨ Types of diarrhoea genic *E. coli*
  1. Enteropathic *E. coli* (EPEC) = diarrhoeas in infants children
     (no toxin production)
  2. Enterotoxic *E. coli* (EEC) = Traveller's diarrhoea = cholera.
  3. Entero invasive *E.coli* (EIEC) = Senery test +ve, = shigella
  4. Enterohaemorrhagic *E. coli* (EHEL) – causes HUS *E. coli* 157,
     H17
  5. Enteroaggressive *E. coli* (EAEL)
⇨ Urease + ve = Klebseilla, protein and Staphylococcus
⇨ Tuberculin test (done with 1TU in India) = ≥ 10 mm = + ve
                                    6-9 mm = doubtful
                                    < 6 mm = – ve
⇨ 3 main tests: Useful for " of TB = heaf test, Tine multipuncture
  test Mantoux's intradermal test
⇨ Gonococci causes (1) water can perineum (2) chronic urethritis
  with stricture formation and (3) ophthalmia neonatorum
⇨ *Cl. tetani* produces 2 toxin = (1) Hemolysin (tetanolysin)
  (2) Neurotoxin (tetanospasmin)
⇨ In presumptive coliform count water is added to " Bile salt lactose
  peptone water"
⇨ Bacteriological examination of milk includes:
  1. Viable count
  2. Test for coliform bacilli
  3. Methylene blue reduction test

4. Examination for specific pathogen
5. Phosphatase test
6. Turbidity test.

⇨ *Staph. aureus* (oil paint appearance of colonies)
Vancomycin = DOC for life-threatening conditions, Topical= Bacitracin

⇨ Streptococcus = Vancomycin = Life-threatening condition
MC streptococcal disease = sore throat (throat culture = Gold standard tests)

⇨ Pneumococcus has somatic C carbohydrate antigen, CRP precipitates with it.

⇨ Commonest pneumococcal infection = otitis media, sinusitis.

⇨ Bacillus Anthracis = Bamboo stick appearance, M'Fadyean's reaction, medusa head appearance.

⇨ Stool is the most diagnostic specimen in acute stage of cholera before administration of antibiotics, on Cary-Blair medium.

⇨ Grading of smear based on number of lepra bacilli
1+ = 1-10 bacilli in 100 fields
2+ = 1-10 bacilli in 10 fields
3+ = 1-10 bacilli in 1 field
4+ = 10-100 bacilli in 1 field
5+ = 100-1000 bacilli in 1 field
6+ = > 1000 bacilli in 1 field

⇨ Citron bodies are formed by clostridium septicum

⇨ Legionella infection = from inhalation of aerosols in air conditioned room at conventions.

⇨ Biological effect of interferones:
1. Antiviral effect
2. Antimicrobial effect
3. Cellular effects
4. Immunoregulatory effects

⇨ Natural evaluation of HIV infections (5 stages)
1. Acute HIV infection (3-6 wks = seroconversion illness)
2. Asymptomatic or latest phase
3. Persistant generalized lymphadenopathy (PGL)
4. AIDS related complex (ARC)
5. AIDS

⇨ Diagnosis of HIV infection (RNA virus)
1. P24 antigen = after 2 wks = earliest method
2. IgM antibody, TgG antibody detection
3. Virus isolation

4. PCR, antibody detection = Gold standard method
5. Western Blot technique

⇨ Retrovirus has RNA dependent DNA polymerase (Reverse transcriptase)

⇨ Double standard DNA containing virus:
- Pox virus
- Papilloma virus (ca cervix)
- Parvovirus has single standard DNA
  (B-19= aplastic crisis in children
- Polioma virus
- Herpes Virus
  - Type 1: HSV1
  - Type 2: HSV2
  - Type 3: V2V
  - Type 4: EBV
  - Type 5: CMV

⇨ Lyophilization of virus = storage of virus

⇨ Pancreatitis = (cancer of pancreas – by clonorchis)

⇨ Romana's sign = Acute Chaga's disease *(T.cruzi)*

⇨ River Blindness = onchocera vulvulus

⇨ Microfilaria are seen in peripheral blood in early adenolymphangiitis stage of filteriasis.

⇨ Hypnozoites are found in *Plasmodium vivax.*

⇨ *Plasmodium vivax* = Schuffner's dots
Plasmodium falispanum = Maurer's dots
Plasmodium ovale = Jame's dots
Plasmodium malariae = Ziemann's dots

Gram + ve = *Cl. tetani*

⇨ Swarming growth

Gram – ve = Proteus mirabilius/vulgaris

⇨ All cocci are gram + ve except Nisseria

⇨ All bacilli are gram – ve except DATTA ⤙ Diphtheria
Actinomycetes
Tetanus cl.
Tuberculosis
mycobacterial
Anthrax bacilli
and listeria
monocytogenes

⇨ Toxins that act by inhibiting protein synthesis
  – Diphtheria toxin
  – Pseudomonas toxin   <u>DPS</u>
  – Shiga toxin
⇨ Hot air oven: glassware, forceps, scissors, scalpels, all glass syringes swabs, liquid paraffin, dusting power, fat, greese.

⇨ **Radiation**

Non ionising: Absorbed as heat: **Infrared radiation**: Rapid mass sterilization of packed item like syringe, catheter: **UV rays**: OT, labs, etc.

Ionizing radiation: Cold sterilization
  – X-ray, gamma ray, cosmic rays
  – Plastic syringes, swabs, catheters animal feeds, carboard, oil, greese, fabrics, metal foils.

⇨ Classification of human herpes viruses (DNA) virus
  Type 1: Herpes simplex type 1
  Type 2: Herpes simplex type 2
  Type 3: Varicella zoster virus
  Type 4: Epstein Barr virus
  Type 5: Cytomegalovirus
⇨ IFNα is produced by leukocytes
  IFNβ is produced by fibroblasts
  IFNγ is produced by T lymphocytes
⇨ EB virus
  — infectious mononucleosis
  — Malignancies
    • Burkitt's lymphoma
    • Nasopharyngeal carcinoma
    • Hodgkin's lymphoma
    • Non-Hodgkin's lymphoma
⇨ Warthus – Finkeldey cells = Measels
⇨ Slow viral diseases:
  – Scrapie
  – Kuru
  – Creutzfeldt = Jacob disease
  – Maedi (sheep) (2-3 yrs)
⇨ Mad cow disease = caused by prions

⇨ Gene coding for structural protein (HIV)
   Gag – determines – core and shell of virus

   Env – determines – envelope glycoprotein gp 160 $\Big\langle$ gp120
    gp 40

   Pol – determines – Viral enzymes (reverse transcriptase, etc)
⇨ Man is intermediate host in:
   • Malaria
   • Cysticercus cellulose
   • Toxoplasma gondii
   • Echinococcus granulosus
⇨ Visceral larva migrans is produced by = Toxocara canis.
⇨ Cutaneous larva Migrans is produced by = Ancylostoma braziliense
⇨ MC cause of Acue Str.endocarditis = staphylococcus
⇨ MC cause of subacute bacterial endocarditis = Streptococcus viridans
⇨ Prozone = zone of antibody excess.

PATHOLOGY

PATHOLOGY

1. PATTERN OF EXAMINATION

PATHOLOGY	Marks
☞ Theory Paper I	40
☞ Theory Paper II	40
☞ Internal Assessment (Theory)	15
☞ Internal Assessment (Prac.)	15
☞ Spotting	5
☞ Slides (Histopathology)	5
☞ Hematological Practical	5
☞ Urine Analysis	5
☞ Viva (Specimen, etc.)	10
☞ Viva (Instruments, etc.)	10
Total	150

Note:

Paper I   * General Pathology
            * Blood
            * Blood vessels
            * Heart

Paper II=   Systemic Pathology

2. QUESTIONS FOR THEORY PAPER

A. QUESTIONS FOR PAPER-1

DW: Hyperplasia and hypertrophy (2005)
DW: Apoptosis and necrosis (2002)
DW: Exudate and transudate (2005)
DW: Caseation and coagulation necrosis
SN: Meningioma (2002)
SN: Familial adenomatous polyposis coli (2002)
DW: Necrosis and autolysis
DW: Dry and wet gangrene
SN: Giant cell tumour of bone (2002)
SN: Prostate specific antigen (2002)
DW: Type II and Type III hypersensitivity reaction (2004)
DW: Hyperplasia and neoplasia
DW: Hyperplasia and hypertrophy
DW: Exudate and transudate (2001)
DW: Dystrophic and metastatic calcification (2001)
DW: Coagulative and liquifactive necrosis
DW: Metastatic and dystrophic calcification
DW: Reversible and irreversible injury
DW: Necrosis and apoptosis
SN: Mixed parotid tumour (2002)
SN: Paget's disease of breast (2002)
DW: Healing by primary and secondary intention
DW: Thrombus and postmortem clot
SN: Hepatitis E (2002)
DW: Labile cell and stable cell
DW: Metaplasia and dysplasia
DW: Granulation tissue and granuloma
SN: Mechanism of CD4 + T helper (2004)
SN: Acute promyelocytic leukemia (2004)
DW: Healing by primary and secondary intentions
DW: Granulomatous inflammation and granulation tissue
DW: Infarction and gangrene
DW: Renal and cardiac edema
DW: T helper and T suppressor cells
SN: Disseminated intravascular coagulation (2004)

SN: Glucose tolerance test (2004)
DW: Class I and class II histocompatibility antigens
DW: T and B lymphocytes
DW: Type I and Type III hypersensitivity reactions
DW: Primary and secondary amyloidosis
DW: Bleeding in platelet and coagulation disorders (2001)
SN: Immune changes in AIDS (2001)
SN: Pathogenesis of hypovolemic shock (2001)
SN: Mechanism of transplant rejection (2001)
SN: Laboratory diagnosis of multiple myeloma (2001)
LQ: Define cell injury. Describe the brief mechanism of hypoxic cell injury
LQ: Describe the process of wound healing by primary intention. What are the factors which influence wound healing
SN: Pancytopenia (2001)
LQ: Define inflammation. Name and discuss the mode of action of chemical mediators in acute inflammation
LQ: Define granuloma, list causes of granulomatosus inflammation, describe the development of tubercular granuloma
SN: Causes of intravascular hemolysis and laboratory diagnosis of Sickle cell anemia (2001)
SN: Spread of tumors (2001)
SN: Klinefelter's syndrome (2001)
DW: Neoplasm and hamartoma
DW: Proto-oncogene and anti-oncogene
DW: Type I and II hypersensitivity
DW: Acute and chronic rejection of renal transplant
DW: Hyaline and amyloid material
SN: Acute radiation syndrome (2004)
SN: Lab diagnosis of chronic renal failure (2004)
DW: Helper and cytotoxic T cells
DW: Ig allotype and idiotype
DW: Benign and malignant tumours
SN: Mechanisms of autoimmune diseases (2001)
SN: Mismatched blood transfusion and its laboratory diagnosis (2001)
SN: Philadelphia chromosome (2001)
SN: Prothrombin time (2001)
DW: Vegetations in SLE and rheumatic endocarditis (2004)

DW: Carcinoma and sarcoma (2001)

DW: Tuberculoid and lepromatous leprosy

DW: Primary and reinfection TB

DW: Kwashiorkar and marasmus

LQ: Discuss pathogenesis of thrombus formation. What is the fate of the thrombus?

LQ: Define and classify shock. Discuss the pathogenesis of endotoxic shock

SN: Prognostic factors of acute lymphoblastic leukemia (2001)

SN: Laboratory findings in chronic renal failure (2001)

LQ: Discuss the etiopathogenesis of thrombosis. Describe the morphology and fate of a thrombus

LQ: Enumerate the different types of edema. Give the pathogenesis of cardiac edema

LQ: Define and classify shock. Discuss the pathogenesis of septic shock

LQ: Define thrombus. Discuss the etiopathogenesis of thrombosis and its fate

DW: Cardiogenic shock and septic shock (2004)

DW: Normoblast and megaloblast (2004)

DW: Iron deficiency anemia and anemia of chronic disease (2004)

SN: Role of human papilloma virus (HPV) in neoplasia (2004)

SN: Chromosomal anomalies and clinical features of Turner's syndrome (2004)

SN: Laboratory diagnosis of megaloblastic anaemia (2004)

SN: Pathogenesis of graft rejection (2004)

LQ: Define hypersensitivity. Describe the mechanism of action of Type II hypersensitivity

DW: Rheumatic and bacterial endocarditis

DW: Vegetations of rheumatic heart disease and bacterial endocarditis

DW: Chronic myeloid leukemia and leukemoid reaction

LQ: Describe the risk factors, pathogenesis and complications of atherosclerosis of aorta

LQ: Classify endocarditis. Describe the etiopathogenesis, pathology and complications of infective bacterial endocarditis

LQ: Enumerate the causes of MI. Describe in brief the pathology and complications of acute MI

LQ: Describe pathogenesis of MI. Give the gross and microscopic features and complications of MI

LQ: Discuss the etiopathogenesis of rheumatic fever. Describe the autopsy findings in the case of mitral stenosis

LQ: Discuss the etiopathogenesis of rheumatic heart disease. Describe the autopsy findings in the case of mitral stenosis

LQ: Describe the gross and microscopic features and lab diagnosis of acute MI

SN: Coomb's test (2004)

SN: Prognostic factors in ALL (2004)

SN: Prothrombin time (2004)

LQ: Enumerate the different types of emboli. Describe the etiopathogenesis and complications of pulmonary embolism

LQ: Classify amyloidosis. Discuss its pathogenesis and characterisation

LQ: Give immunological and clinical classification of amyloidosis. Describe the gross and microscopic autopsy findings in a case of reactive systemic amyloidosis

LQ: Define hypersensitivity. Give pathogenesis of various types of hypersensitivity reactions with examples

SN: Tumour markers and their association with cancer (2004)

LQ: Classify hemolytic anemia. Describe the hematological lab findings in beta-thalassemia

LQ: Classify purpuras. Describe the peripheral blood and bone marrow findings in a case of idiopathic thrombocytopenic purpura

LQ: Classify megaloblastic anemias. Give the pathogenesis and lab diagnosis of pernicious anemia

LQ: Enumerate the causes of iron deficiency anemia. Describe its pathogenesis and lab investigations

LQ: Classify hemolytic anemia. Give the lab diagnosis of B thalassemia

DW: Lepromatous and tuberculoid leprosy (2005)

DW: Acute and chronic ITP (2005)

SN: Down's syndrome (2005)

SN: Lab. diagnosis of hemophilia (2005)

LQ: What are the microcytic anemias. Describe the clinical features and lab diagnosis of iron deficiency anemia

LQ: Define hypersensitivity. Give the mechanism of action of type II hypersensitivity reaction with examples

LQ: Define neoplasia. Describe the altered growth properties of malignant cells and their mode of spread

SN: Mechanism of anaphylactic shock (2005)

SN: Hodgkin's disease (2005)

LQ: Discuss the role of viruses in carcinogenesis. Enumerate the important laboratory techniques used in diagnosis of cancer

LQ: Classify chemical carcinogens. Discuss the sequential steps involved in chemical carcinogenesis

LQ: Define neoplasia. Describe the mechanism of DNA viral carcinogenesis

LQ: Describe briefly the MOA and biological effects of ionising radiations

SN: Apudoma

SN: Hemochromatosis

SN: Pathogenesis of fatty liver

SN: Coagulative and caseous necrosis

LQ: Outline a scheme for investigating a probable patient of hemolytic anemia. Give the pathophysiology and clinical features of beta thalassemia major

LQ: Enumerate the causes of iron deficiency anemia. Describe the hematological findings in a case of nutritional iron deficiency anemia

LQ: Enumerate the viruses implicated in human neoplasia. Discuss the mechanism of action of RNA viruses in inducing neoplastic change

LQ: Classify epithelial tumours and describe the gross and microscopic features of squamous cell carcinoma

SN: Lab anticoagulants

SN: Bone marrow picture of megaloblastic anemia

SN: Disseminated intravascular coagulation (DIC)

SN: Lab diagnosis of sickle cell anemia

SN: Pancytopenia

SN: Hemophilia

SN: Foetal Hb

SN: Erythrocyte sedimentation rate

SN: Hemophilia

SN: Idiopathic thrombocytopenic purpura

SN: Rh incompatibility

LQ: Define carcinogenesis. Describe briefly the role of various carcinogens in causation of human malignancy

SN: Chemical mediators of inflammation (2005)

LQ: Classify leukemias. Describe the clinical features and lab findings in a case of chronic myeloid leukemia

LQ: Describe the salient clinical features, lab findings and prognostic factors of acute lymphoblastic leukemia

LQ: Classify leukemia. Describe the clinical and lab findings in a case of acute myeloid leukemia

LQ: Enumerate the causes of generalised lymphadenopathy in young adults. Describe the gross and microscopic features of Hodgkin's lymphoma

LQ: Classify acute leukemias. Discuss the clinical features, peripheral blood and bone marrow findings in acute lymphoblastic leukemia

SN: Polyarthritis nodosa

SN: Complications of atheromatous plaque

SN: Causes of left ventricular hypertrophy

SN: Constrictive pericarditis

SN: Lab findings in myocardial infarct

SN: Sequelae of bacterial endocarditis

SN: Libman-Sack's endocarditis

SN: Causes and morphological features of vegetations of cardiac valves

SN: Viral myocarditis

SN: Libman-Sacks disease

SN: Constrictive pericarditis

SN: Lab diagnosis of iron deficiency anemia

SN: Blood transfusion reactions

SN: Causes of pancytopenia

SN: G6PD deficiency

SN: Pancytopenia

SN: Prothrombin time

SN: Blood transfusion

SN: Mechanism of platelet destruction in idiopathic thrombocytopenic purpura lab diagnosis of hemophilia

SN: Blood and bone marrow findings in folate deficiency anemia

SN: Lab diagnosis of thalassemia

SN: Peripheral smear changes in megaloblastic anemia

SN: Hemoglobin estimation

SN: Bleeding time
SN: Significance of ESR estimation
SN: Bombay blood group
SN: Hodgkin's disease
SN: β2-microglobulin in multiple myeloma (2005)
SN: Mechanism of amyloid deposition (2005)
SN: Spread of tumours (2005)
SN: Mycotic aneurysm
SN: Thromboangiitis obliterans
SN: Raynaud phenomenon
SN: Sequelae of atherosclerosis
SN: Aneurysms of aorta
SN: Tubercular pericarditis
SN: Pathology of acute MI
SN: Non-bacterial thrombotic endocarditis
SN: Aschoff body
SN: Lab diagnosis of acute MI
SN: Aschoff nodule
SN: Peripheral blood findings in beta-thalassemia major (2005)
SN: Hypercholesterolemia and its significance (2005)
SN: Fibrocongestive spleen
SN: Agranulocytosis
SN: Lab investigation of multiple myeloma
SN: Nodular sclerosing Hodgkin's disease
SN: Histological features of Hodgkin's lymphoma
SN: Peripheral smear and bone marrow findings in chronic myeloid leukaemia
SN: Lab diagnosis of multiple myeloma
SN: Burkitt's lymphoma
SN: Multiple myeloma
SN: Hodgkin's lymphoma-mixed cellularity
SN: Cytochemical differentiation of acute leukaemias
DW: Causes and sequelae of constrictive and fibrinous pericarditis (2002)
SN: Complications of myocardial infarctions (2002)
SN: Dissecting aneurysm (2002)
SN: Etiopathogenesis of disseminated intravascular coagulation (DIC) (2002)
SN: Complications of myocardial infarction (2004)
SN: Acute radiation injury (2005)

SN: Osteomalacia (2005)
SN: Free radical induced injury (2005)
SN: Classification of Hodgkin's lymphoma (2004)
SN: HLA and disease association (2004)
SN: Fat necrosis (2004)
SN: Metastatic and dystrophic calcification
SN: Free radicals in cell injury
SN: Mechanism of fatty change in liver
SN: Mallory's bodies
SN: Causes and morphology of fatty liver
SN: Free radical injury
SN: Dystrophic calcification
SN: Dysplasia
SN: Interleukin-1
SN: Lymphokines
SN: Phagocytosis
SN: Chemotactic factors
SN: Vascular changes in acute inflammation
SN: Granulomatous inflammation
SN: Brown induration of lungs
SN: Fate of thrombus
SN: Phlebothrombosis
SN: Classification and morphology of infarcts
SN: Fat embolism
SN: Amniotic fluid embolism
SN: Venous thrombosis
SN: Paradoxical embolism
SN: Renal oedema
SN: Nutmeg liver
SN: Klinefelter syndrome
SN: Turner's syndrome
SN: Lyon's hypothesis
SN: Glycogen storage disease
SN: Barr body
SN: Hermaphroiditism
SN: Hypercholesterolemia
SN: Acute graft rejection
SN: Staining properties of amyloid
SN: Sago spleen
SN: Type IV hypersensitivity reaction

SN: Interferon
SN: Delayed hypersensitivity
SN: Significance of HLA complex
SN: Coomb's test
SN: Antibody dependent cell-mediated cytotoxicity
SN: Immunologic tolerance
SN: Lab diagnosis of AIDS
SN: Cytokines
SN: Basis of immunodeficiency in AIDS
SN: Opportunistic infection in AIDS
SN: Alfa-fetoprotein
SN: Hazards of radiation
SN: Hemolytic disease of newborn
SN: Neuroblastoma
SN: Hemolytic disease of newborn
DW: Hypertrophy and hyperplasia (2002)
DW: Primary tuberculosis and secondary tuberculosis (2002)
DW: Carcinoma and sarcoma (2002)
SN: Pathogenesis of chronic myeloid leukaemia (2002)
SN: Red infarct (2002)
SN: Etiopathogenesis of amyloidosis (2002)
SN: Pathogenesis of radiation damage and relative radiosen-
     sitivity of tissues (2002)
SN: Significance of microscopic examiantion of urine (2002)
SN: DNA viruses in neoplasia (2002)
SN: Coomb's test (2002)
SN: Haemophilia (2002)
SN: DNA oncogenic viruses
SN: Oncofoetal proteins
SN: Philadelphia chromosome
SN: Alfa-fetoprotein
SN: Role of cytology in tumour diagnosis
SN: Lepromin test
SN: Lepromatous and tuberculoid leprosy
SN: Ghon's complex
SN: Primary complex
SN: Kwashiorkar
SN: Radiation injury
SN: Diet of cancer
SN: G6 PD deficiency (2002)

SN: Hodgkin's disease (2002)
SN: Bombay phenotype blood group (2002)
SN: Role of complement in inflammation (2002)
SN: Carcinoma *in situ*
SN: Tumour cell markers
SN: Role of cytology in early detection of cancer
SN: Procarcinogens
SN: Frozen section
SN: Co-carcinogen
SN: Tumor markers
SN: Teratoma
SN: Cytological diagnosis of cancer
SN: Oncofetal antigens
SN: Indications of bone marrow aspirations (2002)
DW: Necrosis and apoptosis (2006)
DW: Primary and secondary amyloidosis (2006)
DW: Iron deficiency anemia and beta thalassemia trait (2006)
DW: Antemortem thrombus and postmortem clot (2006)
Que: Comment briefly on role of human papilloma virus (HPV) in neoplasia (2006)
Que: Comment briefly on spread of tumour (2006)
Que: Comment briefly on F VIII deficiency (2006)
Que: Write briefly on lab diagnosis of cancer (2006)
Que: Write briefly on pathogenesis of septic shock (2006)
SN: WHO classification of AML and their lab diagnosis (2006)
SN: Laboratory diagnosis of multiple myeloma (2006)
Que: Write briefly on CSF findings in tubercular meningitis (2006)
Que: Write briefly on cytochemistry in acute leukemia (2006)
Que: Write briefly on prothrombin time (2006)
Que: Write briefly on primary complex (2006)
SN: Indications and sites of bone marrow aspiration (2006)
SN: Special stains for Amyloid (2006)
SN: Turner's syndrome (2006)
DW: Rheumatic and infective endocarditis (2006)
DW: Benign and malignant nephrosclerosis (2006)
DW: Tubercular and typhoid ulcer in intestine (2006)
DW: Nephrotic and nephritic syndrome (2006)
Que: Give brief account of laboratory diagnosis of myocardial infarction (2006)

Que: Give brief account of sequelae of rheumatic heart disease. (2006)

DW: Reversible and irreversible cell injury (2007)

DW: Acute and chronic ITP (2007)

DW: Dystrophic and metastatic calcification (2007)

DW: Normoblast and megaloblast (2007)

Que: Comment briefly on lyon hypothesis (2007)

Que: Comment briefly on G6PD deficiency (2007)

Que: Comment briefly on cell mediated hypersensitivity (2007)

Que: Write briefly on paraneoplastic syndrome (2007)

Que: Write briefly on blood component therapy (2007)

SN: Mode of transmission of HIV infection cut throat (2007)

SN: Fate of thrombus (2007)

Que: Write briefly on pathogenesis of septic shock (2007)

Que: Write briefly on pancytopenia (2007)

Que: Write briefly on mechanism of autoimmune disease (2007)

Que: Write briefly on Down's syndrome (2007)

SN: Philadelphia chromosome (2007)

SN: Metaplasia (2007)

SN: Osmotic fragility test (2007)

DW: Healing by primary and secondary intention (2008)

DW: Clonal deletion and Clonal anergy (2008)

DW: Metaplasia and Dysplasia (2008)

DW: CML and Leukemoid reaction (2008)

Que: Comment briefly on laboratory diagnosis of diabetes mellitus (2008)

Que: Comment briefly on Down's syndrome (2008)

Que: Comment briefly on type III hypersensitivity reaction (2008)

Que: Write briefly on pathogenesis of fatty change liver (2008)

Que: Write briefly on component therapy (2008)

SN: DIC (2008)

SN: Laboratory diagnosis of tuberculosis meningitis (2008)

Que: Write briefly on opportunistic infections in AIDS (2008)

Que: Write briefly on laboratory diagnosis of beta-thalassemia (2008)

Que: Write briefly on radiation injury (2008)

Que: Write briefly on factors affecting ESR (2008)

SN: FAB Classification of Acute Myeloid Leukemia (2008)

SN: Mechanics of Apoptosis (2008)

SN: Etiopathogenesis of Shock (2008).

B. QUESTIONS FOR PAPER-2

SN: Mechanism of fatty change in liver (2005)

SN: Etiopathogenesis of gallstones (2004)

DW: Benign and malignant gastric ulcer (2002)

DW: Nephrotic syndrome and nephritic syndrome (2002)

DW: Typhoid and tubercular ulcer (2002)

SN: Diabetic nephropathy (2002)

SN: Endonutrial hyperplasia (2002)

SN: Metastasis of testicular tumours (2004)

SN: Microscopic changes in renal cell carcinoma (2004)

SN: Yolk sac tumour testis (2004)

DW: Renal changes in benign and malignant nephrosclerosis

DW: Features of chronic pyelonephritis and chronic glomerulo-nephritis

DW: Benign and malignant hypertension

SN: Hashimoto's thyroiditis (2002)

SN: Pathogenesis of transitional cell carcinoma bladder (2002)

SN: Krukenberg tumour (2002)

SN: Role of *H. pylori* in gastrointestinal disorders (2002)

DW: Tuberculous and pyogenic pericarditis

DW: Bronchopneumonia and lobar pneumonia

DW: Centriacinar and panacinar emphysema

DW: Features of benign and malignant gastric ulcer

DW: Tubercular and typhoid ulcer intestine

DW: Ulcerative and amoebic colitis

DW: Hepatocellular and obstructive jaundice

DW: Obstructive and hemolytic jaundice

SN: Renal changes in diabetes mellitus (2004)

SN: Glioblastoma multiforma (2004)

SN: Cervical intraepithelial neoplasia (2004)

DW: Chronic glomerulonephritis and chronic pyelonephritis

DW: Minimal changes and membranous nephropathy

DW: Nephroblastoma and renal cell carcinoma

DW: Hydatidiform mole and choriocarcinoma

SN: Burkitt's lymphoma (2004)

DW: Alcoholic and post-necrotic cirrhosis (2002)

DW: Chronic active and chronic persistent hepatitis

DW: Amoebic and pyogenic liver abscess

DW: Hepatitis A and Hepatitis B

DW: Mature and immature teratoma

DW: Follicular carcinoma and papillary carcinoma thyroid

DW: CSF findings in tuberculous and pyogenic meningitis

LQ: What is bronchiectasis? Describe the predisposing factors, pathogenesis morphology and sequelae of bronchiectasis

LQ: Enumerate the causes of hemoptysis. Describe the autopsy findings in a case of fibrocaseous TB lung

DW: Etiopathogenesis of obstructive and hemolytic jaundice (2002)

DW: Pathology of typhoid and tubercular intestinal ulcer (2002)

DW: Hashimoto's thyroiditis and Grave's disease (2002)

SN: Etiopathogenesis of chronic gastric ulcer (2002)

LQ: Classify tumours. Discuss the etiopathogenesis and pathology of squamous cell carcinoma lung

LQ: Enumerate the ulceroinflammatory lesions of small intestine. Describe the pathology and complication of intestinal tuberculosis

LQ: Enumerate the ulceroinflammatory lesions of large intestine. Give the gross and microscopic features and complications of amoebic colitis

LQ: Discuss the etiopathogenesis of peptic ulcer. Describe the pathology and complications of chronic gastric ulcer

LQ: Classify the tumours of stomach. Describe the brief etiopathogenesis, gross and microscopic features of gastric carcinoma

LQ: Discuss the etiology, pathogenesis, pathology and sequelae of acute viral hepatitis

SN: Serological diagnosis of hepatitis C virus infection

SN: Etiopathogenesis and morphology of fibrocongestive spleen (2002)

SN: Bronchogenic carcinoma (2002)

SN: Endometrial carcinoma (2002)

LQ: Classify pneumonias. Describe the etiopathogenesis, pathology and complications of lobar pneumonia

LQ: Describe the primary complex in pulmonary tuberculosis and types of reactivation lesions of the lung and its complications

LQ: What is bronchiectasis. Discuss the pathogenesis, pathological features and complications of bronchiectasis

LQ: Name the cavitating lesions of lung. Describe the gross and microscopic findings in case of longstanding bronchiectasis

LQ: Define bronchiectasis. Describe the predisposing factors, pathogenesis, morphology and sequelae of bronchiectasis

LQ: Classify lung tumours. Discuss the etiological factors for lung cancer and describe the morphology of squamous cell cancer of the lung

LQ: Classify pneumoconiosis. Describe the etiopathogenesis, pathology and complications of silicosis lung

SN: Benign prostatic hyperplasia (2002)

SN: Premalignant lesions of large intestine (2002)

LQ: Classify malignant tumours of the bone. Describe the pathology of a common primary malignant bone tumour

LQ: Describe the etiopathogenesis and gross and microscopic features of chronic osteomyelitis. Enumerate its complications

SN: Emphysema lung

SN: Oat cell carcinoma of lung

SN: Viral pneumonia

SN: Role of alpha-1 antitrypsin in emphysema

SN: Lab diagnosis of bronchogenic carcinoma

SN: Complications of bronchietasis

SN: Asbestosis

SN: Lab diagnosis of bronchogenic carcinoma

SN: Oat cell carcinoma lung

SN: Barrett's esophagus (2002)

LQ: Classify cirrhosis. Discuss brief, the pathology, pathogenesis and complications of posthepatic cirrhosis

LQ: Enumerate the clinical manifestations of cirrhosis of the liver giving the pathological basis of portal hypertension

LQ: Enumerate the viruses that cause hepatitis. Describe the pathology of acute viral hepatitis B and its sequelae

LQ: Define cirrhosis. Describe the etiopathogenesis of post-necrotic cirrhosis and enumerate its complications

LQ: Define and classify cirrhosis. Give the gross and microscopic features of alcoholic cirrhosis

LQ: Define and classify cirrhosis. Describe the pathogenesis and pathology of post-necrotic cirrhosis. Enumerate the complications of post-necrotic cirrhosis

LQ: Enumerate the ulcerative lesions of large intestine. Describe the etiopathogenesis, morphological features and complications of post-necrotic cirrhosis

LQ: Discuss the etiopathogenesis and complications of alcoholic cirrhosis.

SN: Radiological, gross and microscopic picture of osteogenic sarcoma (2002)

SN: Human chronic gonadotropic hormone (2002)

SN: Phyllodes tumor breast (2002)

LQ: What are the types of urinary calculi? Discuss the pathogenesis, gross features and complications of renal calculi

SN: Renal infarct

SN: Benign and malignant hypertension

SN: End stage kidney

SN: Renal changes in DM

SN: Renal changes in malignant hypertension

SN: Urothelial tumours of urinary bladder

SN: Seminoma

SN: Nodular hyperplasia prostate

SN: Seminoma testis

SN: Carcinoma prostate

SN: Hydatidiform mole

SN: Choriocarcinoma

SN: Teratoma ovary

SN: Vesicular mole

SN: Choriocarcinoma

SN: Leiomyoma uterus

SN: Benign cystic teratoma, ovary

SN: Endometrial carcinoma

SN: Uterine cervical intraepithelial neoplasia

SN: Yolk sac tumour

SN: Hydatidiform mole and choriocarcinoma

SN: Cervical intraepithelial neoplasia

SN: Dermoid cyst ovary

SN: Yolk sac tumour of ovary

LQ: Describe the autopsy findings in a 65 years old male who has had DM for 20 years

LQ: Define nephrotic syndrome. Enumerate the causes and discuss its pathogenic mechanism. Describe morphological features of membraneous glomerulonephritis.

LQ: Classify glomerulonephritis. Describe the clinical features, etiopathogenesis and lab diagnosis of post-streptococcal glomerulonephritis

LQ: Describe the pathology and the pathogenesis of acute poststreptococcal glomerulonephritis

SN: Classification of bone tumors and morphology of dysgerminoma (2002)

SN: Paget's disease of the breast

SN: Fibrocystic disease of the breast

SN: Cystosarcoma phylloides

SN: Fibroadenoma breast

SN: Cushing's syndrome

SN: Pheochromocytoma

SN: Thyroiditis

SN: Multinodular goitre.

SN: Pheochromocytoma.

SN: Hashimoto's thyroiditis.

SN: Grave's disease.

SN: Medullary carcinoma thyroid.

SN: Papillary carcinoma thyroid.

SN: Craniopharyngioma.

SN: Adenomatous goitre.

SN: Adenoma thyroid.

SN: Malignant melanoma.

SN: Basal cell carcinoma.

SN: Rodent cancer.

SN: Sequestrum.

SN: Tuberculous osteomyelitis.

SN: Osteoclastoma.

SN: Osteomalacia.

SN: Cephalic index (2006)

DW: Suicidal and homicidal cut throat (2006)

DW: Entry and exit of rifled firearm (2006)

DW: Male and female mandible (2006)

LQ: Define medical negligence. What are the various types of medical negligence along with various precautions a doctor should take to protect against such law suits? (2006)

DW: Antemortem and postmortem drowning (2006)

DW: Dry heat burn and moist heat burn (2006)

SN: Ewing's sarcoma of bone

SN: Bone changes in rickets
SN: Fibrous dysplasia of the bone
SN: Osteogenic sarcoma
SN: Gross and microscopic features of giant cell tumour of bone
SN: Pathogenesis of tuberculous osteomyelitis
LQ: Define nephrotic syndrome. Enumerate its causes, and describe the etiopathogenesis and pathology of membranous glomerulonephritis
LQ: A 55-year-old man died of persistent long standing HT. Discuss autopsy findings
LQ: Describe the etiopathogenesis, morphologic changes and lab findings of chronic pyelonephritis
LQ: Enumerate the cause of thyroid enlargement. Describe the etiopathogenesis and pathology of multinodular goitre
SN: Pathogenesis of bronchial asthma
SN: Viral pneumonia
SN: Complications of lung abscess
SN: Lung abscess
SN: Primary atypical pneumonias
SN: Utility of broncholveolar levage
SN: Alpha-1 antitrypsin deficiency
SN: Complications of bronchiectasis
SN: Pleomorphic adenoma of salivary gland
SN: Pleomorphic adenoma
SN: Coeliac disease
SN: Carcinoid syndrome
SN: Gross and microscopic appearance of amoebic colitis
SN: Hirschprung's disease
SN: Typhoid ulcer of intestine
SN: Complications of ulcerative colitis
SN: Complications of amoebic colitis
SN: Malabsorption syndrome
SN: Crohn's disease
SN: Carcinoid tumour of intestine
SN: Precancerous lesions of GIT
SN: Acute appendicitis
SN: Benign gastric ulcer
SN: Typhoid ulcer
SN: Complications of peptic ulcer
SN: Villous adenoma of colon

SN: Typhoid and tuberculous ulcer of small intestine
SN: Morphological features and complications of ulcerative colitis
SN: Acute appendicitis
SN: Chronic active hepatitis
SN: Indian childhood cirrhosis
SN: Hepatitis B virus
SN: Amoebic liver abscess
SN: Gallstones
SN: Complications of gallstones
SN: Delta hepatitis
SN: Portal hypertension
SN: Non-A non-B hepatitis
SN: Alfatoxin
SN: Lab findings in obstructive jaundice
SN: Mechanism of ascites of cirrhosis of liver
DW: Centriacinar and Panacinar emphysema (2004)
SN: Giant cell tumour of bone (2004)
SN: Sequelae of Hepatitis B (2004)
LQ: Define nephrotic syndrome. Enumerate its causes and describe the renal changes and lab diagnosis of minimal change glomerulonephritis
LQ: Describe etiopathogenesis, clinical features and lab diagnosis of acute proliferative poststreptococcal glomerulonephritis
SN: Zollinger-Ellison's syndrome
SN: Fibrocystic disease of the pancreas
SN: Diabetic neuropathy
SN: Glucose tolerance tests
SN: Ketoacidosis
SN: Diagnostic significance of urinary casts
SN: Amoebic abscess of liver
SN: Morphologic features of alcoholic cirrhosis
SN: Chronic active hepatitis
SN: Hepatocellular carcinoma
SN: Cholelithiasis
SN: Chelating agent (2006)
LQ: Classify neurotic poisons. Describe clinical features, management, postmortem findings and medicolegal significance in a case of datura poisoning (2006)
DW: Poisonous and non-poisonous snake (2006)

SN: Dubin-Johnson's syndrome
SN: Hereditary hyperbilirubinemia
SN: Acute pancreatitis
SN: Acute tubular necrosis
SN: Rapidly progressive glomerulonephritis
SN: Urinary findings in chronic glomerulonephritis
SN: Wilm's tumour
SN: Kidney in hypertension
DW: Laboratory findings in nephritic at nephrotic syndrome (2004)
DW: Ulcerative colitis and Crohn's disease (2004)
SN: Renal infarct
SN: Renal lesions
SN: Benign nephrosclerosis
SN: Urinary casts
LQ: Describe the etiopathogenesis, morphological features and urinary findings in poststreptococcal glomerulonephritis
SN: Rapidly progressive glomerulonephritis
SN: Renal changes in DM
SN: Acute lobar necrosis
SN: Urinary casts
SN: Morphologic lesions of diabetic nephropathy
SN: Malignant nephrosclerosis
SN: Pathogenesis of pyogenic osteomyelitis
SN: Etiopathogenesis of acute pyogenic osteomyelitis
SN: Giant cell tumour of bone
SN: Tubercular osteomyelitis
SN: Rickets
SN: Etiopathogenesis of chronic pyelonephritis (2002)
SN: Osteosarcoma
SN: Pathology and clinical features of chondrosarcoma
SN: CSF findings in acute pyogenic meningitis
SN: CSF in viral meningitis
SN: Astrocytoma
SN: CSF findings in tubercular meningitis
SN: Hydrocephalus
Que: Write briefly on renal stones (2006)
Que: Write briefly on laboratory diagnosis of hepatitis B infection (2006)
Que: Write briefly on Kimmel Steil-Wilson's disease (2006)
SN: Etiopathogenesis of carcinoma colon (2006)

SN: Pathogenesis of alcoholic liver disease (2006)

Que: Write gross and microscopic features of bronchiectasis (2006)

Que: Write gross and microscopic features of chronic pyelo-nephritis (2006)

Que: Write gross and microscopic features of osteogenic sarcoma (2006)

Que: Write gross and microscopic features of colloid goiter (2006)

Que: Write briefly on papillary carcinoma thyroid (2006)

Que: Write briefly on glioblastoma multiforme (2006)

Que: Write briefly on medullary carcinoma, breast (2006)

DW: Tuberculous and amoebic ulcer (2007)

DW: Dilated and hypertrophic cardiomyopathy (2007)

DW: Lobar and bronchopneumonia (2007)

DW: Type I and Type II Diabetes mellitus (2007)

Que: Write briefly on gallstones (2007)

Que: Write briefly on hydatidiform mole (2007)

Que: Write briefly on familial polyposis coli (2007)

Que: Write brief account of ARDS (2007)

Que: Write brief account of etiopathogenesis of emphysema (2007)

SN: Barrett's oesophagus (2007)

SN: Lung abscess (2007)

Que: Write gross and microscopic features of carcinoma prostate (2007)

Que: Write gross and microscopic features of seminoma (2007)

Que: Write gross and microscopic features of meningioma (2007)

Que: Write gross and microscopic features of renal cell carcinoma (2007)

Que: Write briefly on carcinoid syndrome (2007)

Que: Write briefly on causes of portal hypertension (2007)

Que: Write briefly on Krukenberg's tumor (2007)

DW: Nephrotic and Nephritic Syndrome (2008)

DW: Benign and Malignant Gastric Ulcer (2008)

DW: Rheumatic and Bacterial Endocarditis (2008)

DW: Atheroma and Fatty Streak (2008)

Que: Comment briefly on prognostic factors in carcinoma breast (2008)

Que: Comment briefly on clinical features and sequelae of Hepatitis B (2008)

Que: Comment briefly on non-seminomatous germ cell tumors (2008)

Que: Write a brief account of cushing syndrome (2008)
Que: Write a brief account of osteogenic sarcoma. (2008)
Que: Write briefly on hypersplenism and causes of splenomegaly (2008)
Que: Write briefly on cervical intraepithelial neoplasia (2008)
Que: Write briefly on bronchogenic carcinoma (2008)
Que: Write briefly on krukenberg tumor (2008)
Que: Write briefly on barrett esophagus (2008)
Que: Write briefly on Wilms tumour (2008)
SN: Complications of acute myocardial infarction (2008)
SN: Etiopathogenesis and complications of gallstones (2008)
SN: Neuroblastoma (2008).

Note:
LQ: Long Question
SN: Short Note
DW: Difference Between
Que: Question

3. TOPICS FOR SPOTTING

Number of spots—Five spots
1. Bone marrow aspiration needle
2. Lumbar puncture needle
3. Specimen of kidney (amyloidosis)
4. Ileocecal tuberculosis (specimens)
5. Matted lymph nodes
6. Seminoma testis
7. Clinical case (history and questions)
8. Cirrhosis of liver
9. Sago spleen
10. Typhoid ulcer.

4. SLIDES FOR PRACTICAL

1. Fatty liver
2. Amyloidosis kidney
3. Cirrhosis of liver
4. CVC liver
5. Tuberculosis lung
6. Tuberculosis of intestine
7. Thrombus artery
8. Squamous cell papilloma
9. Squamous cell carcinoma skin
10. Lobar pneumonia
11. Bronchopneumonia
12. Fibrocystic disease of breast (FNAC)
13. Duct carcinoma of breast (FNAC)
14. Calloid goitre thyroid (FNAC)
15. Seminoma testis
16. Glomerulonephritis (Acute)
17. Peptic ulcer
18. Lymphadenitis
19. Atheromatous plaque
20. Arteriosclerosis
21. Cavernous hemangioma
22. Lipoma
23. Breast carcinoma
24. Toxic nodular goitre of thyroid
25. Bone tumors.

5. TOPICS FOR HEMATOLOGICAL PRACTICAL

1. Hemoglobin estimation
2. Total leucocyte count calculation methods
3. Differential leucocyte counting method
4. Provisional diagnosis on the basis of:
   - Hb estimation
   - TLC
   - History and results of other investigations provided with blood sample.

6. TOPICS FOR URINE ANALYSIS

⇨ Physical examination of urine:
- Color
- Amount
- Specific gravity
- Odour
- pH
- Transparency, etc.

⇨ Chemical analysis for:
- Protein
- Sugar
- Ketone bodies
- Bile salts
- Bile pigments

⇨ Provisional diagnosis on the basis of:
- History and results of other investigations provided
- Findings after urine analysis of the sample provided.

7. TOPICS FOR THEORY VIVA

⇨ Necrosis
⇨ Inflammation and mediators
⇨ Dry and wet gangrene
⇨ Pathogenesis of edema
⇨ Nutmeg liver
⇨ Sago spleen
⇨ Metabolic/respiratory acidosis
⇨ Metabolic/respiratory alkalosis
⇨ Shock
⇨ Stages of shock
⇨ Pathways of coagulation mechanisms
⇨ Infarction
⇨ Triple response
⇨ Ghon's complex
⇨ Wound healing
⇨ Benign and malignant tumors
⇨ Methods of staging of carcinoma
⇨ Atherosclerosis
⇨ Kaposi's sarcoma
⇨ Left ventricular hypertrophy and right ventricular hypertrophy
⇨ Myocardial infarction
⇨ Pathological changes in MI
⇨ RHD
⇨ Myocarditis
⇨ Laboratory findings in hypochromic and megaloblastic anemia
⇨ Classification of anemia
⇨ Leukemia (ALL and CML)
⇨ Hodgkin's and Non-Hodgkin's lymphoma
⇨ Various types of pneumonia
⇨ Lung abscess
⇨ Pathology of pulmonary tuberculosis
⇨ Emphysema
⇨ COPD
⇨ Pleomorphic adenoma
⇨ Gastric and duodenal ulcers
⇨ Gastric carcinoma

⇨ Crohn's disease and ulcerative colitis
⇨ Intestinal tuberculosis
⇨ Chronic hepatitis
⇨ Amoebic liver abscess
⇨ Cirrhosis of liver
⇨ Features of gallstones
⇨ Polycystic kidney disease
⇨ End stage kidney
⇨ Nephropathy (diabetic and hypertensive)
⇨ Urinary calculi
⇨ Seminoma
⇨ Fibrocystic disease of breast
⇨ Basal cell carcinoma
⇨ Pyogenic osteomyelitis
⇨ Bone tumors (classification)
⇨ Tubercular meningitis
⇨ CSF findings in various types of meningitis
⇨ Limitations of FNAC.

8. IMPORTANT POINTS

A Vegetations on Heart Valves

Rheumatic fever	Non-bacterial thrombotic	Libman Sack's	Infective endocarditis
• Small and irregular	• Small and irregular	• Medium sized	• Large
• Along the line of curvature (MC-under-surface)	• Along the line of curvature	• On surface of cusps	• On upper surface of cusps
• Sterile (Bacteria)	• Sterile	• Sterile	• Non-sterile
• Non-destructive	• Non-destructive	• Destructive	• Ulcerates or Perforates the underlying valve (or myocardium)
• Seen in rheumatic fever	• Seen in hypercoagulable states (cancer, promyelocytic leukemia, etc)	• Seen in SLE	• Seen in infective endocarditis

⇨ Special Types of Cells

	Cells	Location
1.	Peg cells -----------------------	Fallopian tubes
2.	Clara cells --------------------	Bronchial tree (Terminal bronchi)
3.	Kulchitsky cells ------------	Carcinoid tumor
4.	Signet cells ------------------	Krukenberg's tumor
5.	Microglial cells -------------	Brain
6.	Kupffer cells -----------------	Liver
7.	Hurthle's cells --------------	Hashimoto's thyroiditis
8.	Warthin Finkelday cells --	Measels
9.	Tzank cells -------------------	Abnormal keratocytes

⇨ Important Histological Bodies (seen in)

1.	Aschoff body ----------------	Rheumatic fever
2.	Lewy body --------------------	Parkinsonism
3.	Negri body -------------------	Rabies
4.	Heinz body -------------------	G6PD deficiency
5.	Russel body -----------------	Multiple myeloma

6. Psammoma body ---------- Papillary carcinoma of thyroid
   papillary tumor of ovary
7. Councilman body --------- Viral hepatitis
8. Cowdry A body ------------ Herpes infection
9. Mallory hyaline body ----- Alcoholic hyaline
   Indian childhood cirrhosis
   Wilson's disease
   Liver cell carcinoma
10. Ferruginous body ---------- Asbestosis
11. Howell Jolly body --------- Splenectomy
    Megaloblastic anaemia
    Severe hemolytic anemia

⇨ Important Stains

- Fats = Oil Red O
- Glycogen = PAS+ve disatase sensitive
- alpha-1 antitrypsin = PAS + ve disatase resistant
- Iron = Prussian blue
- Hemosiderin = Prussian blue
- Amyloid = Congo Red → bifringes under polarized microscopy
- Calcium = Von Kossa.

⇨ Lymphoma

A group of malignant solid tumors of lymphoid tissue.

Hodgkin's lymphoma (Hodgkin's disease): solid tumors of the lymphoreticular system that can have its origin in any lymphoid tissue, but usually begins in lymph nodes of the supraclavicular, high cervical or mediastinal area.

⇨ Classification (Rye's Classification)

1. Lymphocyte predominant: Good prognosis (Best Prognosis) – Popcorn cells
2. Mixed cellularity - 2nd MC worldwide and MC in India
3. Lymphocyte depletion = Poor prognosis = Least common
4. Nodular sclerosis = Most common = Lacunar cells

Reed-Sternberg cells are found in all types. These are large cells with bilobed nucleus.

⇨ **Staging**

Stage I: One lymph node region involved

Stage II: Involvement of two lymph node regions on one side of diaphragm

Stage III: Lymph node regions involved on both sides of diaphragm

Stage IV: Dissaminated disease with bone marrow or liver involvement:

- Stage A = without symptoms
- Stage B = with symptoms
    1. 10% decrease in Body wt in 6 months
    2. Unexplained fever
    3. Night sweats etc.

Non-Hodgkin's lymphoma: Lymphomas that arise directly from the thymus.

- Low grade lymphomas
- Intermediate grade lymphomas
- High grade lymphomas
- Diffuse large cell NHL is the most malignant form of NHL

Burkitt's lymphoma: A form of malignant Non-Hodgkin's lymphoma that causes bone destroying lesions of the jaw. The Epstein Barr virus is causative agent.

Another classification used is REAL classification, i.e. Revised Europian-American Classification.

⇨ **Renal Stones**

1. **Calcium stones (75%)** = Radiopaque = due to idiopathic hypercalciuria, primary hyperparathyroidism, distal renal tubular acidosis = super saturation of ions in urine, alkaline pH of urine, decreased urine volume.
2. **Struvite (mixed) stones (15%)** = Radiopaque = due to urinary infection with urea splitting organisms like proteus = *alkaline urine* formed by ammonia from splitting of urea by urease.
3. **Uric acid stones (5-6%)** = **Radiolucent** = due to gout, dehydration, malignant tumors, idiopathic= *acidic urine (pH<6)* decreases the solubility of uric acid in urine and favours precipitation.
4. **Cysteine stones (2%)** = Radiopaque(due to sulphur content) = due to genetic defect in cysteine transport = yellow and crystalline stones.

5. **Other types (<2%)** = **Radiolucent** = due to inherited abnormalities of amino acid metabolism = Xanthinuria.

⇨ **Genetic Disorders**

1. *Autosomal:*
   - Patau's syndrome = trisomy of 13th chromosome
   - Edward syndrome = trisomy of 18th chromosome
   - Down's syndrome = trisomy of 21st chromosome, incidence is **1:1000**, *commonest* chromosomal disorder, *mental retardation* is the hallmark of Down's syndrome. Features in newborn include hypotonia, flat facies and dysplastic ears. ALL is more common in Down's syndrome patients.

2. *Sex chromosomal:*
   - **Turner's syndrome** = 45, XO = *single most important cause* of primary amenorrhea in females. Features include broad chest with widely spaced hypoplastic nipples, webbed neck, and increased carrying angle. Abnormalities include horseshoe shaped kidneys, double or cleft renal pelvis, *coarctation of aorta, aortic stenosis,* and perceptive hearing defects.
   - **Klinefelter's syndrome** = 47, XXY = *principle cause of infertility* in males.

True hermaphrodite is an extremely rare condition, both ovarian and testicular tissue is present.

Pseudohermaphrodite is disagreement between phenotypic and gonadal sex:
- Female pseudohermaphroditism, sex is XX, less complex, basis is the excessive and inappropriate exposure to androgenic steroids during early part of gestation
- Male pseudohermaphroditism, presence of Y chromosome, most complex of all disorders of sexual differentiation.

⇨ **Neutrophils** have
   A. Primary granules
      - Appear at promyelocytic stage
      - Contain myeloperoxidase and hydroxylase enzymes
   B. Secondary granules
      - Appear at myelocytic stage
      - Contain lactoferrin, lysozyme and alkaline phosphatase enzymes

⇨ Neutrophils predominate in *early stage* of inflammation (within 24 hours) and macrophages enter *in late stage* (after 24-48 hrs). Neutrophils remain predominant cells up to 72 hrs after which macrophages take over as predominant cells.

⇨ Ketoacidosis is *absent* in malnutrition related diabetes.

⇨ Oncogenes are cancer causing genes derived from proto-oncogenes. Proto-oncogenes are cellular genes that promote normal growth and differentiation.

⇨ Oncogenes encode proteins called oncoproteins, which resemble normal products of proto-oncogenes but they are devoid of important regulatory elements and their production in the transformed cells does not depend on growth factor s or external signals.

⇨ Xanthomas are tumor like collection of foamy histiocytes within the dermis usually the result of impaired secretion of cholesterol and hyperlipidemia.

⇨ **Types of Necrosis**

1. **Coagulative necrosis:**
   - Most common type of necrosis
   - Occurs due to deficient blood supply and anoxia
   - The necrotic cells retain their cellular outline(usually for several days)
   - Typically occurs in solid organs like kidneys, heart, adrenal glands, etc. except brain(Liquefactive necrosis)

2. **Liquefactive necrosis:**
   - Occurs due to liquefaction of necrotic cells by lysosomal enzymes by the necrotic cells
   Examples: Brain following ischemia, suppurative inflammation.

3. **Fat necrosis:**
   a. Enzymatic fat necrosis:
      - Acute pancreatitis
   b. Non-enzymatic fat necrosis (also called traumatic fat necrosis):
      - Cause may be trauma
      Example: Breast, subcutaneous tissue, abdomen.

4. **Fibrinoid necrosis:**
   - Type of connective tissue necrosis

Example: Autoimmune diseases (PAN, SLE, rheumatoid fever), malignant hypertension.

Serum alpha-fetoprotein is a glycoprotein secreted by yolk sac, fetal liver and fetal GIT. Its level is elevated in:

1. Carcinomas
   - Liver carcinoma
   - Colon carcinoma
   - Lung carcinoma
   - Pancreatic carcinoma
   - Non-seminomatous testicular tumors
2. Non-neoplastic conditions
   - Cirrhosis
   - Hepatitis
   - Pregnancy

Macrophages are the phagocytic cells presenting all tissues of body. For example:
   - Brain...............Microglial cells(at the time of injury modify to form *gitter cells*)
   - Liver................Kupffer cells
   - Lung................Alveolar macrophages
   - Lymph follicles....Dendritic cells

⇨ **Complications of Bronchiectasis:**

   - Lung abscess
   - Massive hemoptysis
   - Purulent pericarditis
   - Respiratory failure with chronic cor pulmonale
   - Empyma with or without bronchopleuro fistula
   - Metastatic abscesses in brain, bones, etc.
   - Secondary amyloidosis with nephritic syndrome
   - *NEVER leads to lung carcinoma.*

There are enzymatic and non-enzymatic systems that contribute to inactivation of free radicals

1. Enzymatic systems:
   - Glutathione peroxidase
   - Catalase
   - Superoxide dismutase
2. Non-enzymatic systems (endogenous or exogenous antioxidants)
   - Vitamin E
   - Serum proteins: Albumin, ceruloplasmin, transferring.
   - Sulfhydryl containing compounds: Cysteine and glutathione

Virchow's triad

- Endothelial injury(most important)
- Alteration in normal flow
- Hypercoagulability

⇨ Single most important feature distinguishing benign from malignant tumors is the absence of metastasis

⇨ Grading of tumor is based on degree of differentiation and number of mitoses within the tumor.

⇨ True aneurysms are composed of all layers of the vessel wall, false aneurysms are extravascular hematomas those communicate with the intravascular space (part of vessel wall is missing)

⇨ Atherosclerotic aneurysms usually occur in the abdominal aorta, mostly between the iliac arteries and the iliac bifurcation

⇨ Syphilitic aneurysms occur in tertiary syphilis and are confined to thoracic aorta (ascending aorta and arch of aorta). The tree-bark appearance and cor-bovium are associated with this.

⇨ Hyaline membrane disease is due to deficiency of surfactant (secreted by type 2 pneumocytes). In this there is formation of hyaline membrane composed of fibrin, necrotic epithelial debris and exudative proteins in alveolar ducts and air spaces.

Epidural hematoma

It is a surgical emergency and immediate surgical decompression is required.

- Usually *arterial blood* accumulates between bone and dura.
- Due to rupture of *middle meningeal artery* after trauma.
- Lucid interval of several hours after trauma.
- CT scan shows lens shaped hematoma.

Subdural hematoma

- Venous blood accumulates between dura and arachnoid
- Due to rupture of superficial bridging veins between cortex and sinuses
- Minor trauma may lead to chronic subdurals in alcoholics
- CT scan shows clot.

⇨ Hypertensive intracranial hemorrhage is mostly in putamen, usually due to arteriolar injury

⇨ Subarachnoid hemorrhage is mostly due to rupture of a berry aneurysm.

⇨ In carbon monoxide poisoning bilateral necrosis of globus pallidus occurs

⇨ In methanol poisoning selective bilateral putamenal necrosis occurs

⇨ In chronic ethanol intake Bergman gliosis occurs.

Tumor markers and associated cancers

1. Calcium .... Medullary Ca of thyroid
2. PSA .... Ca prostate
3. CEA .... Adenocarcinoma of colon, pancreas, lung, stomach, breast
4. Ca-125 .... Ca ovary
5. Ca-19-9 .... Ca colon, Ca pancreas
6. Ca-15-3 .... Ca breast
7. Alpha FP and CEA .... Liver cell carcinoma
8. Bence Jones proteins .... Multiple myeloma
9. Alkaline phosphatase .... Ca of bones
10. Alpha FP, beta-HCG, LDH .... Testicular Ca
11. Neuron specific enolase .... Small cell carcinoma of lung
12. Beta-HCG .... Choriocarcinoma, seminoma and non-seminoma of testis

⇨ Beta HCG is increased in both seminoma and non-seminoma of testis but alpha FP is raised only in non-seminomatous testicular tumors.

⇨ Serum alkaline phosphatase (secreted by bones, liver, intestine and placenta) is raised in:
  • Bile duct obstruction
  • Biliary cirrhosis
  • Hyperparathyroidism
  • Infectious mononucleosis
  • Paget's disease
  • Osteogenic sarcoma
  • Metastatic bone tumors
  • Metastatic bone diseases of (rickets, osteomalacia)
  • Pregnancy.

Serum amylase is raised in:

• Perforated peptic ulcer
• Peritonitis

- Diabetic ketoacidosis
- Pancreatitis, cholangiitis
- Chronic liver diseases
- Burns
- Cancer of breast, ovary, lung, esophagus.

Serum LDH is raised in:

- Myocardial infarction
- Renal infarction
- Hepatitis, hepatic metastasis
- Megaloblastic anemia
- Hypoxia, systemic shock.

Associated antigens

- Primary T cell .... CD1 to CD8 (except CD6)
- Primary B cell .... CD10 and CD19 to CD23
- Primary monocyte .... CD13, CD14, CD15 and CD33 (macrophage)
- Primary NK cells .... CD2, CD16 and CD56

Features of reversible cell injury:

- Cellular swelling
- Endoplasmic reticular swelling
- Blebs
- Lipid deposition
- Clumping of nuclear chromatin.

Features of irreversible cell injury:

- Free radicals
- Lipid breakdown
- Increase Ca^{++} in mitochondria
- Nuclear changes
- Protein digestion.

⇨ Metaplasia is a reversible change in which one adult cell type is replaced by another adult cell type (e.g. Barrett's esophagus)

⇨ Cardinal signs of inflammation are **rubor** (redness), **tumor** (swelling), **calor** (heat), and **dolor** (pain).

⇨ **Outcomes of acute inflammation:**

1. Complete resolution
2. Abscess formation
3. Healing by fibrosis
4. Chronic inflammation

⇨ Tissue destruction is the *hallmark* of chronic inflammation.

⇨ Most common mass in anterior mediastinum is *thymoma*.

⇨ Most common mass in middle mediastinum is *congenital cysts* etc.

⇨ Most common mass in posterior mediastinum is *neurogenic tumor*.

⇨ Most common primary cardiac tumor in adults is *myxoma*.

⇨ Most common primary tumor in children is *rhabdomyoma*.

⇨ Myocardial infarction – events:

Elapsed time	Gross or naked eye (at autopsy)	Light microscopic features
0-12 hours	None	• Usually none
12-24 hours	Softening, irregular pallor	• Loss of striations • Cytoplasmic eosinophilic • Nuclear pyknosis • Mild edema
1-3 days	Pale infarct surround by a red (hyperemic) zone	• As above, plus: • Nuclear lysis • More neutrophils • Inflammatory capillary dilatation
4-7 days	Pale or yellow (caused by liquefaction by neutrophils), definite red margin	• As above, plus: • Liquifaction of muscle fibers • Neutrophils • Macrophages remove debris • In growth of granulation tissue from margins
7-14 days	Progressive replacement of yellow infarct by red-purple (granulation) tissue	• As above, plus: • Diappearance of necotic • Reduced numbers of neutrophils • Macrophages, lymphocytes • Beginnings of fibrosis and organisation of granulation tissue.
2-6 weeks	Becomes gray-white	As above, plus: • Development of fibrous scar • Decreasing vascularity • Contraction

FORENSIC MEDICINE

1. PATTERN OF EXAMINATION

FORENSIC MEDICINE	Marks
☞ Theory Paper	40
☞ Internal Assessment (Theory)	10
☞ Internal Assessment (Pract.)	10
☞ Age Report	10
☞ Injury Report	10
☞ Spotting	10
☞ Theory Viva	10
Total	100

2. QUESTIONS FOR THEORY PAPER

A. FORENSIC MEDICINE

DW: Suicidal and homicidal wounds (2004)

SN: Examination-in-chief and cross-examination (2003)

LQ: Discuss in detail the MLI of age

SN: Grievous hurt (2003)

LQ: Enumerate various changes in the body after death. Discuss late changes in detail

DW: Police inquest and Magistrate inquest (2001)

LQ: Enumerate various changes in body after death. How will you determine the time elasped since death?

DW: Suicidal and homicidal cut throat wounds (2001)

LQ: Classify voilent asphyxial deaths. What postmortem findings will help you in deciding the death was due to fresh water drowning?

MLI: Moment of death (2004)

LQ: Define rape. Describe the findings in a case of rape on a 10-years old girl

SN: Priviledged communication (2001)

LQ: Define rape. How will you examine a 12 years old girl who has allegedly been raped? Describe the main findings you expect in such a case

MLI: A patient is doing 'Pill rolling movement' (2003)

LQ: Define rape. Describe the findings in a case of alleged rape in a female of 12 years of age. How would you express your opinion in such cases?

LQ: Define live birth. How will you decide on postmorterm examination whether the infant was born alive or dead

LQ: Discuss in detail about firearm injury

MLI: A child is dead born (2001)

MLI: Contra-coup injuries are present in the head (2001)

SN: Person is an intersex (2001)

SN: Grievious hurt (2001)

DW: Rigor mortis and cadaveric spasm (2001)

DW: Burns and scalds (2001)

LQ: Intracranial hemorrhage

DW: Dying declaration and dying deposition

DW: Documentary and oral evidence

DW: Criminal and civial malpraxis
DW: Male and female femur
MLI: Diatoms present in bone marrow (2001)
DW: Male and female mandible
DW: Male and female sacrum
DW: Causcasoid and negroid skull
DW: Turner's and Klinefelter's syndrome
DW: Male and female sternum
DW: Molecular and somatic death
SN : Adipocere (2001)
DW: Heat stiffening and cold stiffening
DW: Adipocere and mummification
DW: Primary and secondary flaccidity
DW: Incised and incised looking wound
DW: Entrance and exit wound of rifled firearm from close range
DW: Rifled and shotgun firearm catridge
DW: Antemortem and postmortem abrasions
DW: Male and female pelvis (2001)
DW: Postmortem lividity and bruise
DW: Postmortem staining and contusion
DW: True and fabricated bruise
DW: Scald and chemical burns
DW: Antemortem and postmortem blisters
DW: Extradural hemorrhage and heat hematoma
DW: Antemortem and postmortem burns
DW: Ligature marks in strangulation and hanging
DW: Fracture of hyoid bone from hanging and ligature strangulation
DW: Signs of recent and remote delivery
SN : MTP act 1971 (2004)
DW: Superfecundation and superfoetation
DW: Nulliparous and multiparous uterus
DW: Ruptured and fimbriated hymen
DW: True and false virgin
DW: Sadism and masochism
DW: Natural and criminal abortion
DW: Viable and nonviable infant
DW: Illusion and delusion
DW: Psychosis and neurosis
DW: Antemortem and postmortem wounds

DW: Drunkenness and concussion

DW: Suicidal and homicidal firearm wounds

DW: Incised and lacerated wound

DW: Rigor mortis and cadaveric spasm

DW: Magistrate and coroner's inquest

MLI: A child is dead born (2003)

MLI: Girl is of 16 years of age

MLI: Tardien spots are present on postmortem examination

MLI: A person is found dead is having skin poppings

MLI: Body shows cold stiffening

MLI: The dead body showing morbling

MLI: Person is in suspended animation

MLI: Dead body showing postmortem stains on legs, foot and hands

MLI: Defence wounds detected in a person

MLI: Entry wound of shotgun fired from 4 meters

MLI: Firearm is of 12 bore

MLI: Head shows ring fracture of skull

MLI: Body shows heat hematoma

MLI: The body shows pugilistic attitude

MLI: The dead body showing pugilistic attitude

MLI: Death is from mugging

MLI: Death is from immersion syndrome

MLI: Death is from partial hanging

MLI: Death was due to overlying

MLI: Death was a result of "cafe coronary"

MLI: Death is from throttling

MLI: Death was due to traumatic asphyxia

MLI: A female suspected to be a false virgin

MLI: Hydrostatic test is positive

MLI: Bresalau's second life test is positive

SN : Testamehtary capacity (2003)

DW: Animal and human hair (2003)

DW: Male and female pelvis (2003)

DW: Antemortem and postmortem blisters (2003)

LQ: What is intanticide? Describe in detail the postmortem examination of a dead body of a newborn infant brought to you by police (2003)

MLI: Person is suffering from Caffey's syndrome

MLI: Person is suffering from delusions

MLI: Person is suffering from somnolentia
MLI: Accused is suffering from somnabulism
MLI: Foetus is viable foetus
SN : Signs of recent delivery (2003)
SN: Subpnoea
SN: Conduct money
SN: Vicarious responsibility
SN: Informed concent
SN: Nuclear sexing
SN: Gustafson's method of age determination
SN: Adipocere
SN: Cadaveric spasm
SN: Suspended animation
SN: Postmortem caloricity
SN: Laceration
DW: Near range and distant range wounds, caused by rifled firearm (2003)
DW: Abrasion and ant bite marks (2003)
MLI: Skull bone is showing ring fracture (2004)
MLI: Dead body is showing marbling (2004)
MLI: Spalding's sign is positive (2004)
SN: Intracranial hemorrhage
SN: Concussion of the brain
SN: Contercoup injuries
SN: Grievous hurt
SN: Heatstroke
SN: Arborscent marking
SN: Lynching
SN: Sexual asphyxia
SN: Presumptive signs of pregnancy
SN: Bevelling of skull bone is present in case of firearm injury (2003)
SN: Death is due to sexual asphyxia (2003)
MLI: Diatoms are present in bone marrow (2004)
SN: Superimposition (2004)
DW: Human and animal hair (2004)
SN: Masochism
SN: Paederasty
SN: Incest
SN: Sodomy

SN: Changes at umbilicus after birth
SN: Illusions
SN: Mc Naughten's rule
SN: Delirium tremers
SN: Somnambulism
SN: Euthanasia
SN: Lochia
LQ: Define 'Medical negligence'. Discuss the precautions that a physician should take a prevent suits of medical negligence (2004)
DW: True and Feigned insanity (2004)
Que: What are the findings, interpretation and medicolegal importance when death is due to traumatic asphyxia (2006)
Que: What are the findings, interpretation and medicolegal importance when Spalding sign is positive (2006)
Que: What are the findings, interpretation and medicolegal importance when a girl is of sixteen years of age (2006)
Que: What are the findings, interpretation and medicolegal importance when Burtonian's lines are present in a person (2006)
SN: Cephalic index (2006)
SN: Inquest (2006)
LQ: Classify neurotic poisons. Describe clinical features, management, postmortem findings and medicolegal significance in a case of Datura poisoning (2006)
DW: Suicidal and homicidal cut throat (2006)
DW: Entry and exit of rifled firearm (2006)
DW: Male and female mandible (2006)
LQ: Define medical negligence. What are the various types of medical negligence along with various precautions a doctor should take to protect against such law suits? (2006)
DW: Antemortem and postmortem drowning (2006)
DW: Dry heat burn and moist heat burn (2006)
Que: What are the findings, interpretation and medicolegal importance when skull is having a ring fracture (2007)
Que: What are the findings, interpretation and medicolegal importance when body is showing pugilistic attitude (2007)
Que: What are the findings, interpretation and medicolegal importance when person is 12 years of age (2007)

Que: What are the findings, interpretation and medicolegal importance when diatoms are present in bone marrow (2007)

SN: Dying declaration (2007)

SN: Whiplash injury (2007)

SN: Privileged communication (2007)

DW: Burns and scalds (2007)

DW: Antemortem and postmortem contusions (2007)

Que: Define rape. What will be findings in a 15 years old girl alleged to have been raped 12 hours ago? (2007)

SN: Concussion (2007)

SN: DNA fingerprinting (2007)

SN: Impulse (2007)

Que: What are the findings, interpretations and medicolegal importance, when it is stated that hydrostatic test is positive (2008)

Que: What are the findings, interpretations and medicolegal importance, when it is stated that the death is due to traumatic asphyxia (2008)

Que: What are the findings, interpretations and medicolegal importance, when it is stated that cadaveric spasm is present (2008)

Que: What are the findings, interpretations and medicolegal importance, when it is stated that the person is in lucid interval (2008)

SN: Contributory negligence (2008)

SN: True and Feigned mental illness (2008)

DW: Entry arid exit wounds of rifled firearm (2008)

DW: Heat haematoma and extradural haematoma (2008)

DW: Ligature marks of hanging and strangulation (2008)

LQ: Classify thermal injuries. Describe in detail the cause of death, postmortem findings in a case of carbon monoxide poisoning (2008)

SN: Patterned injuries (2008)

SN: Delusion (2008)

SN: Hostile witness (2008).

B. TOXICOLOGY

LQ: Classify systemic poisons. Describe clinical features, management. Postmortem findings and medicolegal significance in a case of chronic lead poisoning (2004)

LQ: What are the various principles of management of a case of acute poisoning. Discuss them in detail

DW: Poisonous and nonpoisonous snakes (2001)

LQ: Classify instant poisons. Discuss symptoms, signs, management and postmortem findings in a case of acute malathion poisoning. What viscera will you preserve for chemical analysis and how?

LQ: Classify irritant poisons. Discuss symptoms, signs, management and postmortem findings in a case of acute sulfur poisoning. What viscera will you preserve for chemical analysis and how?

DW: Colubrine and Viperine bite (2004)

LQ: Classify neurotic poisons. Discuss, symptoms, signs management and postmortem findings in case of acute opium poisoning. What viscera will you preserve for chemical analysis and how?

SN: Contraindication of stomach wash

LQ: What are stupefying poisons? Discuss signs, symptoms, management and postmortem findings in a case of acute datura poisoning

SN: Treatment of poisoning

LQ: What is infanticide? Describe in detail, how you would proceed when the body of a newborn infant has been brought to you by a police officer? (2001)

LQ: Classify neurotic poisons. Discuss, signs, symptoms, management and postmortem findings in a case of acute cyanide poisoning. What viscera will you preserve for chemical analysis and how?

LQ: Classify neurotic poisons. Discuss signs, symptoms, management and postmortem findings in a case of acute carbon monoxide poisoning. What viscera will you preserve for chemical analysis and how?

LQ: Snake poisoning. How will you manage a case of snake bite?

LQ: What is a poison? Discuss in detail how will you proceed for management of a case of unknown poisoning

DW: Stomach changes in sulfuric acid and carbolic acid poisoning

DW: Cholera and arsenic poisoning

DW: Poisonous and nonpoisonous snake

DW: Cobra bite and viper bite

DW: Drug addiction and drug habituation

DW: Tetanus and nux vomica poisoning

DW: Postmortem findings in cyanide and carbon monoxide poisonings

DW: Datura and capsicum seeds

DW: Cobra and viper

LQ: Classify neurotic poisons. Discuss symptoms, signs, management and postmortem findings in a case of acute barbiturate poisoning (2003)

MLI: Person is suffering from caboluna

MLI: Person is suffering from plumbism

MLI: Person is sufferung from erithism

MLI: Person is experiencing cocaine bugs

SN: BAL

SN: Ideal homicidal poison

SN: Ideal suicidal poison

SN: Gastric lavage

SN: Lead poisoning

SN: Plumbism

SN: Delirium tremens

SN: Withdrawal symptoms

LQ: Classify poisons. Describe clinical features, management and postmortem findings in a case of acute cyanide poisoning (2001)

DW: Drug addiction and drug habituation (2004)

DW: Strychnine poisoning and tetanus (2004)

Que: Classify irritant poisons. Describe clinical features, management, postmortem findings and medicolegal importance in a case of chronic mercury poisoning (2007)

DW: Datura and capsicum seeds (2007)

LQ: What are Somniferous poisons? Describe the clinical features, management, postmortem findings and medicolegal significance in a case, of acute morphine poisoning (2008)

Note:

LQ: Long Question

SN: Short Note

MLI: Medicolegal Importance

DW: Difference Between

Que: Question.

3. TOPICS FOR AGE REPORT

Following topics will help you while preparing age report:
⇨ Normal development of male and female child upto 21 years of age.
⇨ Secondary sex characters.
⇨ Pattern of pubic hair in males and females.
⇨ Temporary and permanent teeth.
⇨ Developmental milestones.
⇨ Gustafson's method.
⇨ Appearance and fusion of epiphysis in clavicle scapula.
⇨ Appearance and fusion of epiphysis in femur, tibia, fibula, humerus, radius, ulna, bones of hand, bones of foot.
⇨ Age changes in mandible.

Procedure for Determination of Age

Following particulars should be noted:
1. Name, father's name, age alleged by the person, sex, occupation, address.
2. Date, time, place of examination.
3. Name of the police constable accompanying the person.
4. Marks of identification.
5. Name of the nurse or attendent present at the medical examination.
6. Height and weight.
7. General built and changes of puberty.
8. Radiological examination of the bones.

Note: Opinion about the age should be given based on the findings of physical, dental and radiological examination.

4. TOPICS FOR INJURY REPORT

Following topics will help you while preparing an injury report:
- ➯ Abrasions (with age)
- ➯ Bruises (with age)
- ➯ Lacerations
- ➯ Stab wounds (punctured wounds)
- ➯ Firearms injury (entry wound and exit wound)
- ➯ Types of lacerations
- ➯ Incised wounds
- ➯ Suicidal cut throat marks
- ➯ D/W marks of strangulation, hanging
- ➯ Age of incised wound
- ➯ Wounds from revolvers and automatic pistols.

5. TOPICS FOR SPOTTING

⇨ Gastric lavage tube with funnel
⇨ Ryle's tube
⇨ Ricinus cummunis
⇨ Capsicum annum
⇨ Calotropis
⇨ Snakes
⇨ Opium
⇨ Datura
⇨ Cannabis sativa
⇨ Nerium odorum
⇨ Skull bone
⇨ Knife
⇨ Bullet
⇨ Cartridge of rifled weapon
⇨ Cartridge of shortgun weapon
⇨ Nine months baby (dead)
⇨ File, weapons, sword, chisel, hammer, etc.
⇨ Abrus precatorius
⇨ Spanish fly
⇨ Specimens (wounds)
⇨ Poisons.

6. TOPICS FOR THEORY VIVA

⇨ Definition of forensic medicine
⇨ Medical ethics
⇨ Inquest
⇨ Summons
⇨ Oral evidence
⇨ Types of witness
⇨ Conduct and duties of the doctor in the witness box
⇨ Consent
⇨ Negligence (medical negligence)
⇨ Informed consent
⇨ Gustafson's method
⇨ Animal and human hair
⇨ FDI system of charting teeth
⇨ Preservation of viscera in case of suspected poisoning
⇨ Exhumation
⇨ Somatic death
⇨ Asphyxia
⇨ Classification of postmortem changes
⇨ Rigor mortis
⇨ Putrefaction
⇨ Estimation of postmortem interval
⇨ Abrasion, lacerations
⇨ Ring fracturs of skull
⇨ Stabwound
⇨ Types of firearm
⇨ Cartridge of rifled and shortgun firearm
⇨ Black powder, smokeless powder
⇨ Entry wound and exit wound from firearm weapons
⇨ Point blank
⇨ Whiplasts injury
⇨ Grievous injury
⇨ Filigree burns
⇨ Mechanical asphyxia
⇨ Signs of asphyxia
⇨ Bansdola
⇨ Mugging
⇨ Throttling

⇨ Smothening, gagging, overlying
⇨ Washerwoman's hands
⇨ Sexual asphyxia
⇨ False virgin female
⇨ What constitutes rape
⇨ Rape on virgin (Findings)
⇨ Incest, sodomy, masturbation, sadism
⇨ Sings of live birth
⇨ How will you manage a case of acute poisoning
⇨ Sui
⇨ Fatal period and fatal doses of various poisons
⇨ Snakes
⇨ Identification of poisonous and nonpoisonous snakes.

7. MEDICOLEGAL ASPECT OF FORENSIC MEDICINE

Indian Penal Code (IPC) (1860): Deals with substantive criminal law of India. It defines offences and prescribes punishments.

CRIMINAL PROCEDURE CODE (Cr. P.C.) (1973)

It provides the mechanism for punishment of offences against the substantive criminal law. It formulates police duties and in investigating offences.

INDIAN EVIDENCE ACT (I.E.A) (1972)

It is common to both the criminal and civil procedures.

IMPORTANT Cr. P.C. LIST (TOTAL Cr. PCs = 484)

1. *S 174 Cr. P.C.:* Officer-in-charge of a police station conducts the inquest except in Mumbai.
2. *S. 28 Cr. P.C.:* An assistant sessions court can pass any sentence authorised by law except a sentence of death or imprisonment for a term exceeding 10 years.
3. *S.41 Cr. P.C.:* In non-cognisable offences, the injuried person may file an affidavit in the court of a magstrate who will send him to the doctor for examination and report.
4. *S. 29 Cr. P.C.:* Powers of magistrate

	Imprisonment	Fine
a. Chief Judicial Magistrate =	< 7 years	yes
b. I class Judicial Magistrate =	< 3 years	Rs. 5000.00
c. II class Judicial Magistrate =	< 1 year	Rs. 1000.00

5. *S. 95 Cr. P.C.:* A summon must be obeyed and the witness should produce documents if asked for.

IMPORTANT I.P.C. LIST (TOTAL IPCs = 511)

1. *S. 118 I.P.C.:* Councealing design to commit offences punishable with death or imprisonment for life.
2. *S 176 I.P.C.:* Omission to give notice or information to public servant by person legally bound to give it.
3. *S. 177 I.P.C.:* Furnishing false information.
4. *S 178 I.P.C.:* Refusing oath or affirmation when duly required by public servant to make it.

5. *S. 179 I.P.C.:* Refusing to answer public servent authorised to question.
6. *S. 182 I.P.C.:* False information with intent to cause public servant to use his lawful power to the injury of another person.
7. *S. 191 I.P.C.:* Giving false evidence.
8. *S. 192 I.P.C.:* Fabricating false evidence.
9. *S. 193 I.P.C.:* Punishment for false evidence.
10. *S. 194 I.P.C.:* Giving or fabricating false evidence with intent to produce conviction of capital offence.
11. *S. 195 I.P.C.:* Giving or fabricating false evidence with intent to produce conviction of offence punishable with imprisonment for life or imprisonment.
12. *S. 197 I.P.C.:* Issuing or signing false certificate.
13. *S. 201 I.P.C.:* Causing disappearance of evidence of offence or giving false information to screen offenders.
14. *S. 2030 I.P.C.:* Giving false information respecting an offence committed.
15. *S. 204 I.P.C.:* Destruction of document to prevent its production as evidence.
16. *S. 87 I.P.C.:* A person above 18 years of age can give valid consent to suffer any harm which may result from an act not intended or not known to cause death or grievous hurt.
17. *S. 88 I.P.C.:* A person can give valid consent to suffer any harm which may result from an act, not intended or not known to cause death, done in good faith and for its benefit.
18. *S. 89 I.P.C.:* In case of child under 12 years of age, consent of the parent or guardian should be taken.
19. *S. 90 I.P.C.:* The consent given byn an insane or intoxicated persone, who is unable to understand the nature and consequences of that to which he gives his consent is invalid.
20. *S, 52 I.P.C.:* Nothing is said to be is good faith which is done without due care and attention.
21. *S. 82 I.P.C.:* Any act done by child under seven years of age is not an offence.
22. *S. 83 I.P.C.:* A child between 7-12 years is persumed to capable of committing an offence, if he attained sufficient maturity of understanding to judge the nature and consequence of his conduct on that occasion.

23. *S. 375 I.P.C.:* Sexual intercourse by a man with a girl under 15 years of age even if she is his own wife, or with any other girl below 16 years of age even with her consent is rape.

24. *S. 369 I.P.C.:* To kidnap a child with the intention of taking dishonestly, any movable property, if the age of child is < 10 years.

25. *S. 361 I.P.C.:* To kidnap a minor from lawful quardianship if the age of boy is < 16 year and girl < 18 years.

26. *S. 366A I.P.C.:* To procure a girl for prostitution if her age is < 18 years.

27. *S. 366B I.P.C.:* To import into India from a foriegn country a female for purpose of illict intercourse if she is belows 21 years of age.

28. *S. 44 I.P.C.:* Defines injury. An injury is any harm, whatever illegally caused to any person in body, mind, reputation or property.

29. *S. 300 I.P.C.:* Defines murder.

30. *S. 299 I.P.C.:* Culpable homicide.

31. *S. 304 I.P.C.:* Imprisonment for life or upto 10 years and also fine.

32. *S. 304A I.P.C.:* Rash or negligent homicide punishment.

33. *S. 302 I.P.C.:* Death, or imprisonment for life and punishment for murder.

34. *S. 319 I.P.C.:* Defines hurt = Bodily pain disease or infirmity causes to any person.

35. *S. 320 I.P.C.:* Defines grievous hurt which is as follows:
    1. Permanent privation of sight of either eye.
    2. Permanent privation of hearing of either ear.
    3. Privation of any member or joint.
    4. Destruction or permanent impairing of the power of any member or joint.
    5. Permanent disfiguration of head or face.
    6. Fracture or dislocation of a bone or tooth.
    7. Any hurt which endagers life, or which causes the victim to be in severe bodily pain or unable to follow his ordinary persuits for a period of 20 days.

36. *S. 323 I.P.C.:* Punishment for voluntarily causing hurt = Imprisonment upto one year or fine upto Rs. 1000 or both.

37. *S. 324 I.P.C.:* Voluntarily causing hurt by dangerous weapons or means = upto three years or fine or both.

38. *S.325 I.P.C.:* Punishment for voluntarily causing grievous hurt = upto seven years with fine.

39. *S. 326 I.P.C.:* Punishment for voluntarily causing grievous hurt by dangerous weapons or means upto 10 years + fine.

40. *S. 351 I.P.C.:* Defines assault = An assault is an offer or threat or attempt to apply force to body of another in a hostile manner.

41. *S. 304 B.I.P.C.:* Dowry death.

42. *S. 498 I.P.C.:* Whoever being the husband or the relative of the husband of the women, subject such women to cruelty shall be punished with imprisonment < three years and/or fine.

43. *S. 396 I.P.C.:* Punishment of rape.

8. SOME IMPORTANT POISONS

	Poison	Fetal dose	Fetal period	Antidote
1.	Copper	15 gm	1-3 days	• EDTA, BAL
2.	Abrus precatorius	90-120 mg	3-5 days	• Antirabin injection
3.	Opium	2 gm opium 0.2 gm morphine	6-12 hrs	• Naloxone hydrochloride
4.	Datura	0.6-1 g	24 hrs	• Physostigmine
5.	Nux Vomica	15-50 gm crusted seeds	1-2 hrs	• Pentobarbital sodium
6.	Nerium odorum	15-20 gm root	24-36	• Symptomatic treatment
7.	Aconite	1-2 gm root or 1-2 mg of aconite	2-6 hrs	• Atropine

9. SOME IMPORTANT DIFFERENCES (SOLVED)

1. Dying Declaration	Dying Deposition
• It is recorded by police, doctor or by any another person, if there is time, magistrate should be called to record the statement	• It is always recorded by magistrate
• Not recorded in presence of accused or lawer (who happen to be present)	• Recorded in presence of his or her lawer
• Victim is not cross examined leading questions can be asked if any point is not clear	• Cross-examination is allowed
• Evidential value is less	• Evidential value is more
• Declaration is recorded in words of victim	• Not necessary, Magistrate draws conclusion and then records
• Verbal statements are also recorded as such	• Conclusion is recorded
• This method is followed in India	• This method is not follwed in India

2. Documentary Evidence	Oral Evidence
• It includes medical certificate medical certification of death and medicolegal reports	• Includes all statements which the court permits or which are required to be made before it by the witness
• Accepted in court only when they are issued by a qualified registered medical practitioner	• Not so
• It is usually indirect	• It must be direct
• It does not permit cross-examination	• It permits cross-examination
• Less important than oral evidence	• More important than documentary evidence
• These are accepted in court only on oral testimony by the person concerned	• Produced in court by the witness himself/herself
• Description of material things, etc. are already present in documentary evidence	• Court may require the production of material thing, referred by oral evidence, for inspection
• Some exception of oral evidences are produced as documentary evidence	• Evidence, e.g. dying declaration, public, records, hospital records, etc are exception to oral evidence

3. Male Femur	Female Femur
• Head is larger and forms about 2/3rd of a sphere	• Head is smaller and forms less than 2/3rd of a sphere
• Vertical diameter of head is more than 47 mm	• Vertical diameter of head is less than 45 mm
• Neck has obtuse angle with shaft (about 125°)	• Neck has less obtuse angle with shaft
• Bicondylar width = 74-89 mm	• Bicondylar width= 67-76 mm
• Angulation of shaft with condyles is around 80°	• Angulation of shaft with condyles is around 76°

4. Male Mandible	Female Mandible
• Generally longer and thicker	• Generally smaller and thinner
• Chin is square	• Chin is rounded
• Body height is greater at symphysis	• Body height is smaller at symphysis
• Breadth of ascending ramus is greater	• Width of ascending ramus is smaller
• Angle of body and ramus is less obtuse (<125°), prominent and everted	• Angle of body and the ramus is more obtuse, not prominent and inverted
• Condyles are larger	• Condyles are smaller

5. Male Sacrum	Female Sacrum
• It is larger	• It is shorter
• It is narrower	• It is wider
• It has more evenly distributed curvature	• Upper half is almost straight curve forword is lower half
• Sacral promontory is well marked	• Sacrum promontary is less marked
• Body of first sacral vertebra is larger	• Body of first sacral vertebra is smaller

6. **Male Sternum**	**Female Sternum**
• Body is longer	• Body is smaller
• Body length is more than twice the length of manubrium	• Length of body is less than twice of the length of manubrium
• Upper margin of sternum is in the level with lower part of body of second thoracic vertebra	• Upper margin of sternum is in the level with lower part of body of third thoracic vertebra
• Breadth is more	• Breadth is less
• Length is more than 149 mm	• Length is less than 149 mm

7. **Turner's Syndrome**	**Klinefelter's Syndrome**
• Anatomical structure = Female	• Anatomical structure = Male
• Genotype - 45, XO	• Genotype = 47, XXY
• Nuclear sexing = male	• Nuclear sexing = female
• It is due to monosomy of X chromosome	• It is due to non-disjunction at the time of meosis in one of the parents.
• Incidence is more than Klinefelter syndrome	• Incidence = one in 850 live male births
• Diagnosed at birth by edema of dorsum of hands and feed, bone skin folds in nape of neck, loose birth wt and short strature	• Diagnosed when there is delay in onset of puberty behavioural disorder and mental retardation
• *Characterised by:* Primary amenorrhea, sterility lack of development of primary and secondary sexual characters webbed neck, wide-set nipples, high arch palate, low-set ears, slow growth, coarctation of aorta, septal defect and renal defect and ovaries do not contain primordial follicles	• *Characterised by:* Absence of pubic or axillary hairs reduced hairs on chest and chin Gynaecomastia, azoospermia. Low level of testosterone sterility and testicular atrophy with hyalinization of seminiferous tubules

8. Molecular Death	Somatic Death
• It is also called as cellular death	• It is also called as systemic or clinical death
• It is the death of cells and tissue individually	• It is the complete and irreversible stoppage of circulation, respiration and brain function
• It occurs after 1-2 hours the stoppage of viral function	• It occurs as soon death occurs
• Death once occurred is irreversible	• Death can be reversed by resuscitation and organ transplant
• Death depends on metabolic activity of the cell, e.g. nervous tissue die in 5 min while muscles die in 1-2 hours	• Usually all the vital functions are lost simultaneously

9. Heat Stiffening	Cold Stiffening
• It occurs where body is exposed to temperature > 65°C	• It occurs when body is exposed to freezing temperature
• Rigidity is produced	• Tissue become frozen and stiff
• Degree and depth of change depends on the intensity of the heat and time for which it was applied	• Degree of change depend on time for which body was exposed and how low was the surrounding temperature
• Heat causes stiffening of the muscles, because the tissue proteins are denatured and coagulated as in cooking	• Freezing of the body fluids and solidification of subcutaneous fat occurs
• Change is much more marked than that found in rigor mortis	• Change is less marked than heat stiffening
• A zone of brownish-pink cooked meat is seen overlying normal red muscle	• No clear demarcation
• Irreversible, i.e. charge do not disappear at normal temperature	• Reversible: When body is placed in warm environment the stiffness disappears after some time
• Normal Rigor mortis does not occur	• Normal rigor mortis occurs

10. Adipocere	Mummification
• In this the fatty tissue of body change into a substance called adepocere	• In this dehydration and drying and shrivelling of cadaver occurs from the evaporation of water
• It is first formed in the subcutaneous tissue usually face, buttock, breast and abdomen are usual sites	• Begins in exposed parts of body like face hands and feet and then extends to entire body including the internal organs
• Change is due to gradual hydrolysis and hydrogenation of pre-existing fat which combine with Ca^{++} and NH^{4+} to form insoluble, soaps	• Change is due to dehydration or drying of tissues and shrivelling by evaporation of water
• There is no weight loss body remains as such, i.e. does not become thin	• The entire body becomes thin, looses weight, stiff and brittle
• Time required = three weeks to six months	• Time required = three months to one year

• Factos contributing to formation
  • Heat
  • Water
	• Factors contributing to formation
	  1. Absence of moisture in air
	  2. Continuous action of dry/warmed air

• If not attacked by animals adepocere may persist for years	• If a mummified body not protected it will break into several fragments gradually, become powdery and disintegrate

11. Primary Flaccidity	**Secondary Flaccidity**
• During this death is only somatic and lasts for 1-2 hrs	• During this death is molecular and flaccidity is permanent
• All body muscles begin to relax soon after death	• Muscles relax after rigor mortis is over
• Muscular irrtability and response to mechanical or electrical stimuli persists	• Muscular irritability and response to mechanical and electrical stimuli is absent
• This occurs due to stomatic death	• It occurs due to break-down of actinomycin due to putrefaction
• Pupils react to atropine or physostigmine	• Pupils do not react to atropine or phyostigmine
• Anaerobic chemical process may continue in the tissue cells, e.g. liver cells may dehydrogenate ethyl alcohol to acetic acid	• No anaerobic process occurs in tissue
• Muscle protoplasm is slightly alkaline	• Protoplasm of muscles again become alkaline

12.

Rifled Cartidge	Shotgun Cartidge
• Length is less	• Length is 5-7 cm
• Usually have not wad	• It contains wad which acts as a piston and seals the bore completely prevent the gases from escaping and disturbing the shot.
• It contains a single bullet	• It contains several pallets
• Muzzle velocity= 450-1500 m/sec	• Muzzle velocity= 240-300 m/sec
• Bullet as it leaves the barrel rotates at speed = 3000 rev/sec	• Does not rotate
• Can kill at a range of upto 3000 metre	• Effective upto 30-35 metre
• Cannot produce tattooing	• Produce tattooing and blackening
• Produce smaller entrance wound	• Produce larger (in case of contact shot) or multiple entrance wounds
• Produce single exit wound	• Usually do not produce exit wound if produce (in contact shot) then very big
• High penetrating power	• Less penetrating power

10. IMPORTANT POINTS

A. VARIOUS CHANGES IN THE BODY AFTER DEATH

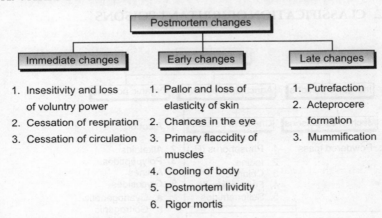

Postmortem changes

Immediate changes	Early changes	Late changes
1. Insesitivity and loss of voluntry power	1. Pallor and loss of elasticity of skin	1. Putrefaction
2. Cessation of respiration	2. Chances in the eye	2. Acteprocere formation
3. Cessation of circulation	3. Primary flaccidity of muscles	3. Mummification
	4. Cooling of body	
	5. Postmortem lividity	
	6. Rigor mortis	

B. VOILENT ASPHYXIAL DEATHS

1. Hanging
    i. Accidental hanging
    ii. Suicidal hanging
    iii. Homicidal hanging
    iv. Lynching
    v. Judicial hanging
2. Strangulation
    i. Homicidal strangulation
        a. Strangulation by ligature
        b. Bansdola
        c. Garrotting
        d. Mugging
    ii. Accidental strangulation
3. Throttling
4. Suffocation
5. Smothering
6. Gagging
7. Overlaying
8. Burking
9. Choking
10. Cafe coronary

11. Traumatic asphyxia
12. Drowning
13. Sexual asphyxia.

C. CLASSIFICATION OF IRRITANT POISONS

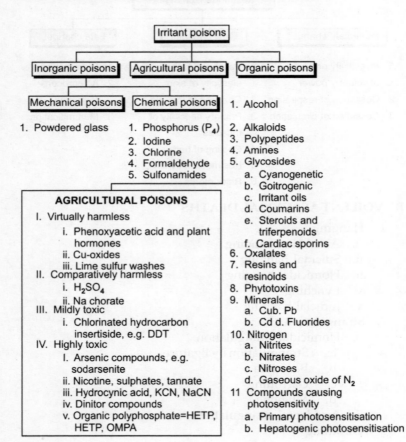

```
                        Irritant poisons
                              |
        ┌─────────────────────┼─────────────────────┐
  Inorganic poisons    Agricultural poisons    Organic poisons
        |
 ┌──────────────┐
Mechanical poisons   Chemical poisons        1. Alcohol
```

Mechanical poisons

1. Powdered glass

Chemical poisons

1. Phosphorus (P_4)
2. Iodine
3. Chlorine
4. Formaldehyde
5. Sulfonamides

Organic poisons

1. Alcohol
2. Alkaloids
3. Polypeptides
4. Amines
5. Glycosides
   a. Cyanogenetic
   b. Goitrogenic
   c. Irritant oils
   d. Coumarins
   e. Steroids and triferpenoids
   f. Cardiac sporins
6. Oxalates
7. Resins and resinoids
8. Phytotoxins
9. Minerals
   a. Cub. Pb
   b. Cd d. Fluorides
10. Nitrogen
    a. Nitrites
    b. Nitrates
    c. Nitroses
    d. Gaseous oxide of N_2
11 Compounds causing photosensitivity
    a. Primary photosensitisation
    b. Hepatogenic photosensitisation

AGRICULTURAL POISONS

I. Virtually harmless
   i. Phenoxyacetic acid and plant hormones
   ii. Cu-oxides
   iii. Lime sulfur washes
II. Comparatively harmless
   i. H_2SO_4
   ii. Na chorate
III. Mildly toxic
   i. Chlorinated hydrocarbon insertiside, e.g. DDT
IV. Highly toxic
   I. Arsenic compounds, e.g. sodarsenite
   ii. Nicotine, sulphates, tannate
   iii. Hydrocynic acid, KCN, NaCN
   iv. Dinitor compounds
   v. Organic polyphosphate=HETP, HETP, OMPA

D. NEUROTIC POISONS

1. CNS Depressants
   - i. Ethyl alcohols
   - ii. General anaesthetics
   - iii. Opioids analgesics
   - iv. Sedative hypnotics
     - a. Barbiturates
     - b. Benzodiazepines
     - c. Nonbarbiturate
     - d. Alcohols
     - e. Propanediol carbamate
     - f. Piperidinediones
     - g. Quinazolines
2. CNS Stimulants
   - i. Tricyclic
     - a. Tertiary amines: Immipramine
     - b. Secondary amines: Nortryptiline.
   - ii. Tetracycline: Maprotiline.
   - iii. Dibenzoxazepine: Amoxapine.
   - iv. Trizolpridine: Trazodone.
   - v. Bicyclic: Fluoxetine.
3. Spinal Poisons
   - i. Strychine.
4. Peripheral Nerve Poisons
   - i. Curare.
   - ii. Conium maculatum.

AGRICULTURAL POISONS

- I. Virtually harmless
  - i. Phenoxyacetic acid and plant hormones
  - ii. Cu-oxides
  - iii. Lime sulfur washes
- II. Comparatively harmless
  - i. H_2SO_4
  - ii. Na chlorate
- III. Mildly toxic
  - i. Chlorinated hydrocarbon insectiside, e.g. DDT

IV. Highly toxic
    i. Arsenic compounds, e.g. sodium arsenite
    ii. Nicotine, sulphates, tannate
    iii. Hydrocynic acid, KCN, NaCN
    iv. Dinitor compounds
    v. Organic polyphosphate = HETP, HETP, OMPA

⇨ Age of an abrasion
(exact age cannot be determined)
- Fresh = Bright red
- 12-24 hr = Bright Scab
- 2-3 days = Redish Brown Scab
- 4-7 days = Epithelium grows and covers defect under scab
- after 7 days = Scab circles, Shrinks and falls off.

⇨ Age of Bruise
- Fresh = Red (24 hrs)
- Few hrs to 3 days = Blue
- 4th day = Bluish Black and Brown (Hemosiderin)
- 5-6 days = Greenish (Haematoidin)
- 7-12 days = Yellow (Bilirubin)
- 2 weeks = Normal

⇨ Hair:
1. Human Hair = fine and thin, thick cortex, narrow medulla.
2. Animal Hair = coarse and thick, thin cortex, wider medulla.
3. Caucasian = Interrupted pattern = occasional breaks in medulla.
4. Fetus and some newborn = Fragmented type = only sporadic medullary structure are seen, Most of the shaft being Non-Medulla feel.
5. Negroid, Mongoloid = Discontinuous type.
Uniform Medulla
Denie pigment irregular

⇨ Davidson body = used to determine sex

⇨ Ashley's rule:

Length of sternum
$\begin{cases} < 149 \text{ mm} = \text{Female adult} \\ > 149 \text{ mm} = \text{Male adult} \end{cases}$

⇨ Ischio pubic index $= \dfrac{\text{Pubic length (mm)}}{\text{Ischial length (mm)}} \times 100$

$$= \begin{cases} \text{Male} = 73\text{-}94 \\ \text{Female} = 91\text{-}115 \end{cases}$$

⇨ For Age determine $\begin{cases} 13\text{-}16 \text{ yr} = \text{X-ray of elbow joint} \\ 16\text{-}25 \text{ yr} = \text{Elbow, wrist and shoulder joint (X-ray)} \end{cases}$

⇨ Length of fetus:

Age	length (cm)
• End of 5th Month	= 25
• End of 6th Month	= 30
• End of 7th Month	= 35
• End of 8th Month	= 40
• End of 9th Month	= 45
• End of 10th Month	= 50-52

⇨ **IQ**

	Mental retardation
0-20 = Idiot	• Mild = 50-70 (IQ)
20-50 = imbecile	• Moderate = 35-50
50- 70 = Moron	• Severe = 20-35
	• Profound = < 20

⇨ Types of abrasion:
1. Scratches
2. Grazes (MC type)
3. Pressure abrasion
4. Impact abrasion
   = Contact or imprint abrasion
   = Patterned abrasion

⇨ Types of lacerations:
1. Split laceration (incised looking wound)
2. Stretch laceration
3. Avulsion
4. Tears
5. Cut lacerations

⇨ Wounds from shot guns
- Smoke = up to 30 cm
- Burnt powder and grains = 60-90 cm
- Flame = 45 cm
- Contact shot
- Close range = upto 1 m
- Near range = upto 4 m
- Long Range = > 4m

⇨ Wounds from revolvers and automatic pistals
- Smoke = 30 cm
- Burnt powder and grain = 60-90 cm
- Flame = 8 cm
- Contact shot = 5-8 cm
- Near shot = upto 60 cm
- Distant shot > 60 cm

⇨ Dumdum bullet: is open at base and has the point covered with jacket. When it strikes an object, the lead of the point expands or mushrooms and produces large hole.

⇨ Black gun powder has
1. Charcoal 15%
2. Sulphur 10%
3. Pot nitrate 75%

⇨ Smokeless powder
Blackgun gun powder + Nitrocellulase or nitroglycerine

⇨ Filigre burns = Seen in lightning, Jule Burn = Electric Burn

⇨ Crocodile skin effect = Very high voltage electric burn

⇨ Test for stoppage of circulation:
1. Magnus test
2. I card test
3. Diaphanous test

⇨ Surest sign of hanging = Saliva running out of mouth (antemortem hanging)

⇨ Malingening (shamming) = conscious planned feinging or pertaining a disease for the shake of gain.

⇨ Jevenile = boy <16 yr, girl <18yrs

⇨ Period of stay in Jevenile home should not exceed beyond 18 yr of age of girl.

⇨ 5.304-B-IPC = Dowry death.

⇨ Indecent Assault is punishable under 5.354 IPC

⇨ Countercoup lesions = Lesion is present is an area opposite to site of impact.

⇨ MC form of traumatic intracranial hemorrhage = subarachnoid hemorrhage

⇨ Scold = Injury which results from application of liquids above 60°C or from steam.

⇨ Common methods of Homicidal strangulation
1. Bansdola with bamboo or sticks
2. Strangulation by ligature
3. Garrotting (attacked from behind)
4. Throttling = with hands = Manul strangulation
5. Mugging = Holding the neck of victim in bend of elbow.

⇨ Death appears to be due to sudden heart attack in café coronary (cause = asphyxia)

⇨ Types of drawning:
1. Wet drawning
2. Dry drawning: Water does not enter lung. Death results from immediate sustained laryngeal spasm due to in thrush of water in nasopharynx or larynx
3. Secondary drawning = Near drawning
4. Immersion syndrome = Death result due to cardiac arrest due to vagal stimuli

⇨ Incest = Sexual intercourse by a man with a woman who is closely related to him by blood (sister)

⇨ Sodomy = anal sex = gerontophilia = with adults
= paederasty = with Young boy (catamite)
= pedophile = with Children

⇨ Tribadism = Lesbianism = Female homosexuality

⇨ Bestiality = Sexual intercourse by a human with lower animal

⇨ Sadism = Sexual gratification is obtained Or increased by physical cruelty or infliction of pain upon one's partner

⇨ Lust murder = extreme case of sadism is lust murder

⇨ Masochism = opposite to sadism = sexual gratification is obtained by suffering of pain.

⇨ Necrophilia = desire for intercourse with dead bodies.

⇨ Transvestism or eonism = Personality of a person is dominated by the desire to be identified with the opposite sex.

⇨ Thanatology = Deals with death in all its aspects.

⇨ Postmortem changes:

    I. Immediate (Somatic death)

       1. Insensibility and loss of voluntary power

       2. Cessation of respiration

       3. Cessation of circulation

    II. Early changes (Cellular death)

       1. Pallor and loss of elasticity of skin within few minutes.

       2. Changes in eye

       3. Primary flaccidity of muscles = starts soon after death and lasts up to 1-2 hrs

       4. Cooling of body (Algor mortis) = ½ -1 hrs later → uniform slope of ↓ temperature.

       5. Postmortem lividity (Liver Mortis) = Begins soon after death, evident = 6 hrs

       6. Rigor mortis = begins 1 – 2 hrs after death and takes further 1-2 hrs to develop duration = 24-48 hrs (winter), 18-36 hrs (summer).

    III. Late changes

       1. Putrefaction = begins soon after death at cellular level, which is not evident grossly

          → Colour changes = 12-18 hr (summer) 24-48 hr (winter)

          → Development of foul smelling gas = 18-36 hr or 48 hr after death.

       2. Adipocere formation = Gradual hydrolysis and hydrogenation of pre-existing fat. Shortest time = 3 wk 1 is summer, it may persist for years decades.

       3. Mummification = Time required for complete mummification = 3 months to 1 year.

⇨ Prostate and virgin uterus are last organs to putrefy
⇨ Poisons that retard putrefaction = Arsenic, antimony, Zinc chloride, datura, strychnine (Nux Vomica) Endrin.
⇨ Cadaveric spasm = is cases of sudden death, fear or excitement, severe pain, exhaustion, cerebral haemorrhage, firearm wound of head, convulsant poison like strychnine.
⇨ Mechanism of rigor mortis:

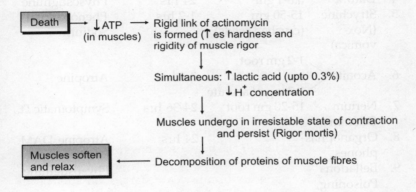

⇨ Levels of consciousness:
    Grade 0: Fully conscious
    Grade 1: Drowsy but respond to verbal command.
    Grade 2: Maximum response to minimum painful stimulus
    Grade 3: Minimum response to maximal painful stimulus
    Grade 4: No response to painful stimulus.

	Poison	Fetal dose	Fetal period	Antidose
1.	Copper	15 gm	1-3 days	EDTA, BaL
2.	Abrus Precatorim	90-120 mg (Inj)	3-5 days	Antirabin (Inj)
3.	Opium	2 gm opium or 0.2 gm morphins	6-12 hrs	Naloxone
4.	Datura	0.6-1 gm	24 hrs	Physostigmine
5.	Strychine (Nox-vomica)	15-50 gm (crushed seeds)	1-2 hrs	Phenobarbital Sodium
6.	Aconite	1-2 gm root or 1-2 mg of aconite	2-6 hrs	Atropine
7.	Nerium Odonim	15-20 gm root	24-36 hrs	Symptomatic Tt.
8.	Organophas-phones		24 hrs	Atropine, DAM, PAM
9.	Belladons Poisoning, atronine			Physostigmine
10.	Arsenic			Freshly prepared hydrated Ferric oxide (alternative dialygodirum)

⇨ Run amoke = caused by canbis = has THC (9-Tetrahydro-cannibol)
⇨ Widmark's formula is used in estimation of alcohol.
⇨ Cocaine bugs = Magnan's syndrome = seen in cocaine poisoning.
⇨ Arsenic poisoning = Mee's lines seen, Marsch's test
  Antidote = Freshly prepared hydrated ferric oxide
⇨ Preservation of viscera in case of suspected poisonings.
  1. Stomach and its contents
  2. Upper part of small intestine (~ 30 CM)
  3. Liver (~ ½)
  4. Kidney = (½ of each or 1)

5. Blood (30 ml, min 10 ml)
6. Urine = 30 ml.

⇨ Carboluria = Urine in carbolic acid poisoning turns green or even black on standing.

⇨ 10 D's of Datura (sign and symptoms)
1. Delirium
2. Dryness of mouth
3. Dysarthria
4. Dysphagia
5. Dilation of pupils
6. Dry hot skin
7. Diplopia
8. Drunken gait
9. Drowsiness
10. Death

Antidote: Physostigmine

⇨ Universal antidote has (1) Activated charcal (2) Magnesium oxide and (3) Tannic acid.

⇨ Marqui test = Done for morphine poisoning.

⇨ Ideal homicidal poison = organic compound of fluorine and thallium, e.g. example: rodenticide, AS and aconite are commonly used.

⇨ Ideal suicidal poisons: Opium, barbiturates; organophosphorus compounds and endrins are commonly used.

⇨ Phossy jaw = seen in poisoning with white phosphorus.

⇨ Features of poisonous snakes
1. Small head scales (large with pit → Pit viper)
2. Large belly scales which cover the entire breath
3. Hypodermic needle like teeth (2 fangs)
4. Compressed tail
5. Usually nocturnal

⇨ Examples of poisonous snakes
– Cobra
– King cobra
– Common krait
– Russel viper
– Saw scaled viper
– Sea snakes

⇨ Non-poisonous snake
– Rat snakes

⇨ Neurotoxic toxins = Cobra krait coral

⇨ Vasculotoxic toxins = Viper

⇨ Myotoxic toxins = Sea Snake

⇨ Test for seminal fluid
   1. Florence test
   2. Barberio test
   3. Acid phosphatase test
   4. Creatinine phosphokinase test

⇨ Tests for blood
   1. Benzidine test
   2. Luminol test
   3. Haemin crystal test
   4. Hemochromogen crystal test

⇨ Test (chemical) for blood stains:
   1. Phenolphthalein test
   2. Orthotolidine test

⇨ Embalming is the treatment of the dead body with antiseptics and preservatives to prevent putrefaction.

⇨ Haemodialysis is not useful in poisoning with
   1. Kerosin oil
   2. Digitalis
   3. BZD
   4. Organophosphates

⇨ Preservative for 10 ml blood in poisoning with Alcohol is mixture of
   1. Potassium oxalate = anticoagulant
   2. NaF = Enzyme inhibitor

⇨ Test for determining criminal responsibility.
   1. MC Naughten's role
   2. Durham rule
   3. Curren's rule
   4. Irrestible impulse test
   5. American law institution test

⇨ Pupils:
   A. Dilated in poisoning with:-
      A^4 = Atropine, Alcohol, Amphetamines, Tricyclic antidepressants
      B = Belladone
      C^3 = Cocaine, cannabis, calotropis
      D = Datura

F^2 = Ergot, endrin

S = Strychnine (Nux Vomica)

B. Contracted pupils in poisons with

P = Phenol

E = Ethanol

P = Physostigmine

N = Nicotine

O^2 = Opium, organophosphorus

B = BZD

C. Alternate contraction and dilation = Hippus = Aconite poisons

⇨ Colour of lividity in poisoning:
- Carbon Monoxide—Bright cherry red
- Potassium cyanide—Pink
- Potassium Chlorate—Chocolate brown
- Nitrites—Red brown
- Hydrogen sulphide—Bluish green
- Opium—Black

⇨ Indication for antivenum therapy after snake bite
1. Rapidly progressive and severe local findings (soft tissue swelling, ecchymosis, petechiae, etc.)
2. Manifestation of systemic toxicity.

Mummification	Adipocere
• It is modification of process of putrefaction	• Is a modification of the process of putrefaction
• Is characterized by- Dehydration or desiccation of body tissues and vicera after death	• It is characterized by conversion of fatty tissues into fatty acids resulting in formation yellowish white greasy wax like substance with a rancid smell
• The body looses moisture and desiccate	
• Ideal conditions includes:	• The body gains moisture and undergoes hydrolysis (of fat into fatty acid) and hydrogenation
– high atmosphere temperature	
– devoid of moisture	• Ideal conditions include:
– free circulation of air around body	– warm temperature
	– moisture
	– relative dimunition of air
	– Bacteria and fat splitting enzymes

	Blacks (Negroes)	Europeans	Mongols
Cephalic index	70-74.9	75-79.9	80 or above
Height index	72	71	75
Nasal index	55	46	50
Orbits	Square	Triangular	Rounded
Nasal opening	Broad	Narrow and elongated	Rounded
Palate	Rectangular	triangular	Rounded or horseshoe shaped

VENOM

Neurotoxic	*Vasculotoxic*	*Myotoxic*
Examples: – Cobra – Krait – Coral	Vipers	Sea snake
• Venom causes muscular weakness of legs and paralysis involving muscles of face	• Venom causes enzymatic destruction of cell walls and coagulation disorders	• Venom produces generalized muscular pain followed by myoglobinuria, three to five hrs later ending in respiratory failure
• Acts on motor nerve cells and resembles curare	• Acts on endothelial cell of blood vessels and red cells are lysed – Haemolysis	
• Local symptoms at site of bite are minimum	• Local symptoms at site of bite are severe – Severe swelling, oozing of blood and cellulitis	
• Cobra venom produces convulsions and paralysis while Krait venom produces only paralysis		

DIFFERENCE BETWEEN POISONOUS AND NON-POISONOUS SNAKES

		Poisonous	Non-poisonous
1.	Belly scales	• Large and cover the entire breadth of the belly	• Small like those on the back or moderately large but do not cover the entire breadth of the belly
2.	Head scales	• Small • Large and with a. Conspicuous pits between the eye end nostrile (pit vipers) b. Third labial touches the eye and nasal shields (Cobra, King cobra or coral) c. Central row of scales on back enlarged and under surface of the mouth with only four infralabial, the fourth being the largest (kraits) and perhaps with bands or half ring across the back	• Large
3.	Fang	Long and grooved or canalized	Short and solid
4.	Tail	Compressed	Not markedly compressed
5.	Habits	Generally nocturnal	Not so
6.	Bite	Two fangs marks with or without small marks of other teeth	A number of small teeth marks in a row

APPENDICES

APPENDIX 1

PROFORMA FOR HISTORY TAKING

1. **BIODATA**
   - Name, age and sex
   - Address and occupation
   - Marital status.
2. **PRESENTING COMPLAINTS**
   - In chronological order.
3. **HISTORY OF PRESENTING ILLNESS**
   - Onset, duration, progression
   - Specific events
   - Negative history.
4. **PAST HISTORY**
   - History of similar disease
   - History of DM, TB, HT
   - Any relevant disease.
5. **HISTORY OF ALLERGY AND DRUGS**
   - Allergy to drugs (specify)
   - Other allergies
   - Long-term drug intake.
6. **PERSONAL HISTORY**
   - Food and bowel habits (normal/abnormal)
   - Sleep
   - Addictions — Yes-specify / No
   - Menstrual and obs history in case of female patient.
7. **FAMILY HISTORY**
   - History of similar disease
   - History of DM, TB, HT, heart diseases
   - History of genetically transmitted diseases.

APPENDIX 2

PROFORMA FOR GENERAL PHYSICAL EXAMINATION

1. • **Built** (Avg/tall/short stature)
   • **Nutrition** (Average/undernurished)
   • **Decubitus** (sitting/lying, comfortably/uncomfortably in bed).
2. **Pallor** (Present/absent) [Sites: (1) Nailbed, (2) lower palpebral conjunctive, (3) mucous membrane of lips and cheeks, (4) Palmer surface of hands].
3. **Cyanosis** ($<$ Present Absent $<$ Central Peripheral) [Sites: (i) Nailbed, (2) tip of nose, (3) tongue, (4) skin of palm and soles].
4. **Jaundice** (Present/not present) [Sites: (1) Nailbed, (2) sclera of eyeball, (3) tip of none, tongue, (4) lobule of ear].
5. **Clubbing** [not present/present (grades)].
6. **JVP** (Raised/not raised).
7. **Edema** [Present (type)/not present]
8. **Lymphadenopathy** [Present / Localised, Not present / Generalised]
9. **Vitals**
   a. **Pulse**
      • Rate (beats per min) (Normal/Bradycardia/Tachycardia)
      • Rhythm (Regular/irregular)
      • Character (normal/abnormal)
      • Volume (average/low/good).
   b. **Temp**
      • °F
      • Site (Axillary/Oral/Rectal)
      • Febrile/Afebrile to touch if the thermometer is not available.
   c. **Respiration**
      • Rate (normal ↑, ↓)
      • Rhythm (regular/irregular)

- Type
  Thoracoabdominal—normal in Females
  Abdominothoracic—normal in Males
- Thoracic
- Abdominal

d. **Blood pressure**
   - ....mm Hg
   - Artery (Brachial/Femoral)
   - Position of the patient (supine/sitting, etc.).

10. **General Survey**
    1. Skin = Normal/Abnormal (findings).
    2. Nail = Normal/Abnormal (specify).
    3. Hair = Quantity, colour, texture, any abnormal finding.
    4. General survey of whole body palpate for any spine tenderness, sternal tenderness, etc.

IMPORTANT POINTS

1. **CAUSES OF LONG (TALL) STATURE**
   1. Genetic.
   2. Hyperpituitarism.
   3. Hypogonadism.
   4. Klinefelter syndrome.
   5. Marfan's syndrome.

2. **CAUSES OF SHORT STATURE**
   1. Delayed growth.
   2. Insulin deficiency.
   3. Hypopituitarism and hypergonadism.
   4. Turner's and Down's syndrome.
   5. Malnutrition/malabsorption.

3. **HYPOPROTEINEMIA CAUSES**
   1. Rough skin.
   2. Brittle hair.
   3. Edema.

4. **FAT MALNUTRITION CAUSES**
   1. Cachexia.
   2. Hollowing of cheeks.
   3. Loss of shape of hip and ↓ fat on other sides.

5. **DECUBITUS IS CHANGED IN**
   1. Pneumonia and pleurisy.
   2. Colic.
   3. Meningitis and tetanus.
   4. Acute abdomen.

6. **CAUSES OF PALLOR**
   1. Anaemia.
   2. Shock and syncope.
   3. Iron deficiency → anaemia → pallor.
   4. Raynaud's disease.
   5. PVD (Peripheral vascular disease).

7. **CAUSES OF CYANOSIS**
   A. *Central*
      1. Congenital cyanotic heart disease.
      2. CHF (Congestive heart failure).

3. COPD.
4. Collapse and fibrosis of lung.

B. *Peripheral*
   1. Cold ($\Rightarrow$ local vasoconstriction $\rightarrow$ cyanosis).
   2. $\uparrow$ viscosity of blood.
   3. Shock and heart failure.

C. *Combined*
   1. Acute left ventricular failure.
   2. Mitral stenosis.

8. **CAUSES OF RISE IN JVP (N^M = 3-4 CM)**
   1. $\uparrow$ in blood volume.
   2. Cardiac tamponade.
   3. Asthma and emphysema.
   4. Tricuspid stenosis.
   5. Superior vena cava obstruction.
   6. Rt ventricular failure.

9. **CAUSES OF JAUNDICE**

A. *Prehepatic*
   1. Sickle cell anaemia and thalassemia.
   2. PNH.
   3. Malaria, quinine and sulfonamides.
   4. Burns and snake venum.
   5. Mismatched blood transfusion and SLE.
   6. Cirrhosis of liver.

B. *Hepatic*
   1. Viral hepatitis.
   2. Malaria, typhoid, antitubercular drugs.
   3. Septicemia.
   4. Cirrhosis, DDT, Gold, Hg.

C. *Posthepatic*
   1. Biliary atresia, stricture, stone.
   2. Acute cholecystitis.
   3. Cholecystic phase of intestive hepatitis.
   4. Carcinoma of head of pancreas.
   5. Steroids, sulfonamides, methyltestosterone.

10. **CAUSES OF CLUBBING**
    1. C—Crohn's disease, congenital cyanotic heart disease, cirrhosis of liver.
    2. L—Lung abscess and TB.

3. U—Ulcerative colitis.
4. B—Bronchogenic carcinoma.
5. B—Bronchiectasis.
6. I—Idiopathic.
7. N—Inf. endocarditis and SABE.
8. G—Grave's disease.

11. CAUSES OF EDEMA
1. Disturbances in renal function (nephritis/nephrosis).
2. Congenital heart failure, LVF, pericarditis.
3. Cirrhosis of liver and portal HT.
4. ↓ plasma proteins, anaemia, malnutrition.
5. IVC/lymphatic obstruction.
6. Inflammation/allergy (Angioneurotic edema).
7. Fluid and electrolyte disturbance (particularly Na^+ retention).

GENERALISED EDEMA

Cirrhosis of liver
Nephrotic syndrome
Severe CHF
Severe nutritional hyporoteinemia

12. CAUSES OF UNILATERAL EDEMA
1. Lymphatic obstruction.
2. Traumatic = Bruises/fractures, etc.
3. Intective = cellulitis, boils.
4. Gout.
5. Venous thrombosis, varicose and veins.

FACIAL EDEMA: FNAC MTV

F   Facial trichinosis.
N   Nephrotic syndrome.
A   Angioneurotic edema.
C   Constructive pericarditis.
M   Myxoedema.
T   Tricuspid valve disease.
V   Vena cava obs (superior).

13. CAUSES OF LYMPHADENOPATHY
1. Acute lymphadenitis.
2. Sarcoma, carcinoma, malignant melanoma.
3. Septic, lymphogranuloma inguinale.
4. TB/syphilis/filariasis.

5. Drug reaction, SLE, serum sickness rheumatoid arthritis.
6. Hodgkin's/non-Hodgkin's lymphoma.
7. Other causes.

14. CAUSES OF HYPOTHERMIA
1. Hypothyroidism.
2. Exposure to cold.
3. Hypoglycemia.
4. Alcoholic intoxication, barbiturate poisoning, ketoacidosis.

15. CAUSES OF FEVER
A. *Fever with Rigor*
   1. Malaria, kala azar, filariasis.
   2. UTI.
   3. Septicemia and inf. endocarditis.

B. *Fever with Herpes Labialis*
   1. Pneumonia.
   2. Streptococcal infection.
   3. Meningitis.
   4. Malaria.

C. *Fever with Rash*
   1. Rubella.
   2. Allergy.
   3. Typhoid.
   4. Chickenpox.
   5. Smallpox.
   6. Measles.

D. *Fever with Membrane in Throat*
   1. Moniliasis.
   2. Agranulocytosis.
   3. Infectious mononucleosis.
   4. Diphtheria.

E. *Fever with delirium*
   1. Pneumonia.
   2. Meningitis.
   3. Typhoid.

F. *Other Causes of Fever*
   1. Bact/viral/fungal infection.
   2. Heatstroke, radiation sickness, crush injury.
   3. Neoplasm, MI, TB.
   4. Gout, acidosis.

16. CAUSES OF HYPERPYREXIA (>105°F)
1. Heatstroke.
2. Pontine hemorrhage.
3. Encephalitis.
4. Malaria.
5. Tetanus.
6. Septicemia.

17. SLOW RISING PULSE IS SEEN IN AORTIC STENOSIS

18. BISFERIENS PULSE IS SEEN IN AORTIC STENOSIS/ INCOMPETENCE

19. COLLAPSING PULSE IS SEEN IN
1. Severe anaemia.
2. Aortic reg.
3. Thyrotoxicosis.

20. PULSUS PARADOXUS IN
1. $\downarrow\downarrow$ BP.
2. Severe asthma.
3. Pericardial effusion.
4. CHF.

21. PULSUS ALTERNANS IS SEEN IN CASE OF SEVERELY DISEASES VENTRICLE

22. CAUSES OF DELIRIUM
1. Cerebral malaria.
2. Alcohol.
3. Renal failure.
4. Typhoid.

23. CAUSES OF DELUSIONS
1. Mania.
2. Schizophrenia.
3. Depression.

24. CAUSES OF PORTAL HYPERTENSION
1. Portal vein thrombosis.
2. Venoocclusive disease.
3. Residual heart failure.
4. Budd Chiari syndrome.
5. Hepatocellular carcinoma.
6. Postal/hepatic fibrosis.

7. Cirrhosis of liver/constructive pericarditis.
8. Acute appendicitis/peritonitis.
9. Pregnancy and oral contraceptives.

25. CAUSES OF ASCITES

1. Pancreatic ascites.
2. Spontaneous bact peritonitis.
3. Meig's syndrome.
4. Portal HT.
5. Severe heart failure.
6. Malignant ascites.
7. Filariasis.
8. Nephrotic syndrome.
9. Anaemia and tuberculosis.
10. Constructive pericarditis.

26. ASCITES + PLEURAL EFFUSION IN

1. Tuberculosis.
2. Meig's syndrome.
3. Pancreatic ascites.
4. Heart failure.

27. CAUSES OF HYPERTENSION

1. Atherosclerosis/coarctation of aorta.
2. Renal A Stenosis.
3. Polycystic kidney.
4. Aortic incompetence.
5. Raised intracranial tension.
6. Toxaemic of pregnancy.
7. Glomerulonephritis.
8. Idiopathic (essential).
9. Thyrotoxicosis.

28. COMPLICATIONS OF HYPERTENSION

1. Coronary A disease.
2. Aneurysm of aorta.
3. Renal insufficiency/failure.
4. TIA = treatment ischemic attack.
5. Cerebral thrombosis.
6. Hypertensive retinopathy/encephalopathy.
7. Angina pectoris.
8. Left ventricular failure.

OTHER PROFORMAS FOR FURTHER EXAMINATION OF PATIENTS

1. RESPIRATORY SYSTEM EXAMINATION

INSPECTION

(1) CHEST WALL

⇨ Shape (normal/abnormal)
⇨ Skin and surface (Scars veins, pulsation, shiny skin, etc.)
⇨ Chest diameter (Transverse: AP:: 7: 5 as normal ratio)
⇨ Epigastric angle
  • Normal = 70-110°
  • ↓ or ↑, specify
⇨ Spine = curvature (normal/abnormal), movements.

(2) RESPIRATORY MOVEMENTS

• Rate = (normal = 14-18 per min)
• Rhythm normal = Regular, normal ration of insp:Exp is 2:3
  Abn = irregular (specify)
• Character type or
  Normal Thoracoabdominal = in ?
  Abdominothoracic = in ?
  Abnormal = thoracic, abdominal
• Symmetry and depth (normal/abdominal on both sides)
• Respiration to pulse ratio (normal = 1:4)
• Use of accessory muscle of respiration or not (muscles = SCM, scaleni, Trapezius, ala nasi)
• Any intercostal retraction with inspiration and bulging with expiration (+/-).

(3) MEDIASTINUM

• Trail sign (+/-)
• Apex impulse (visible or not).

PALPATION

⇨ Chest wall = tenderness (+/-), other findings of inspection

⇨ Chest movements = symmetry (+/-) • expansion of chest (normal = 1.5-2 inches)

⇨ Trachea (Central/deviated to one side)

⇨ Apex impulse (palpate/not palpable)

⇨ TVF (normal, ↓,↑)

⇨ Misc = Laryngeal fixation, palpable rales, rhonchi, etc.

PERCUSSION

⇨ Anteriorly
  • Right side = Liver dullness, tidal percussion, shifting dullness
  • Left side = Cardiac dullness, shifting dullness, traube's area.

⇨ Posteriorly = Suprascapular, interscapular and infrascapular region.

⇨ Axilla = Upper, middle and lower axilla.

AUSCULTATION

⇨ Breath sounds (normal/abnormal, specify type (vesicular/ bronchial).

⇨ Vocal resonance (normal, ↓,↑ also specify side of chest when ↑ or ↓).

⇨ Other sounds = Rhonchi, rales, crepitation fine course pleural rub, etc.

⇨ Misc: coin test, succussion splash, etc, wherever applicable.

2. CARDIOVASCULAR SYSTEM EXAMINATION

INSPECTION

⇨ Shape of chest wall   (normal/abnormal)

⇨ Precordium = shape (normal = smooth, slightly convex and symmetrical with the part of chest wall on opp. side) (Abnormal = findings (flattened/bulging, etc.)

⇨ Apex impulse = visible/not Normal/shifted (specify)

⇨ Other pulsations = • epigastric, supracentral, left parasternal, etc.

⇨ Scars (+/-), sinus (+/-), dialated veins (+/-), ulcers (+/-), etc.

PALPATION

⇨ Apex beat = (+/-), side, heaving/tapping apex (+/-)

⇨ Left parasternal heave (+,-)

⇨ Diastolic shock (palpable S2) (+/-)

⇨ Thrills (+/-) other pulsations (+/-).

PERCUSSION

⇨ Heart borders

(i) Right border = retrosternal.

(ii) Left border = along apex beat vertically.

(iii) Upper border = in between 2nd and 3rd I/C space.

(iv) Lower sternal resonance.

AUSCULTATION

⇨ Heart sounds = • Intensity, • Picth, • Quality, • Splitting (First heart sound and second heart sound)

⇨ Murmurs (+/-) =   • Site and timing
                       • Intensity
                       • Quality and pitch
                       • Radiation and grading

⇨ Other sounds
   • Opening snap • Ejection clicks • pericardial rub, etc.

3. GASTROINTESTINAL TRACT EXAMINATION

EXAMINATION OF ORAL CAVITY

1. Lips [normal/abnormal (findings)].
2. Gums (normal/any swelling/bleeding), etc.
3. Teeth (colour, shape, ridging, caries, any missing tooth, etc).
4. Tongue (colour, moistness, fur papillae).
5. Buccal mucosa (normal/Abnormal—findings).
6. Tonsils (enlarged/not enlarged).
7. Oropharynx (normal/Abnormal—findings).

EXAMINATION OF ABDOMEN

A. INSPECTION

1. Shape (normal/abnormal)
   normal = flat
   Abnormal = Globular, scaphoid, uniform distention, irregular distention.
2. Abdominal movements
   i. With respiration (normal = free and equal on both sides
      (Males) = Abdominothoracic
      (Females) = Thoracoabdominal.
   ii. Any other movements (pulsation, etc).
3. Skin and surface
   - Prominent veins (+/-)
   - Pulsations (+/-)
   - Peristalsis (+/-)
   - Scars (+/-)
   - Sinus (+/-)
   - Pigmentation (+/-)
   - Ulcer (+/-)
   - Umbilicus
     Normal = Retracted and inserted
     Abnormal = Findings
   - Hernial orifices (inguinal, femoral, epigastric, umbilicus) (normal/abnormal).

B. PALPATION

1. Tenderness (+/-), Guarding (+/-), Rigidity (+/-).
2. Edema (+/-), Fluid thrill (+/-).

3. Visceral organs = liver (+/-). spleen (+/-), kidneys (+/), gallbladder (+/-) and urinary bladder (+/-) .
4. If any lump is present then note its
   - Local temperature and tenderness
   - Perital or intra-abdominal
   - Edge, margin and consistency
   - Movements (i) with respiration
                (ii) Up down
                (iii) Sideways.

C. PERCUSSION

(i) Shifting dullness
(ii) Over organs and lump (if any)

D. AUSCULTATION

(i) Peristalsis (+/-)
(ii) Bruit, rub, etc.
(iii) other abnormal sounds appreciated
Misc: (i) PR, (ii) PV, Proctoscopy.

4. CENTRAL NERVOUS SYSTEM EXAMINATION

EXAMINATION OF HIGHER MENTAL FUNCTIONS

1. Orientation to time person and place (+/-).
2. Consciousness = (fully conscious/semiconscious/drowsiness/stupur/coma).
3. Behaviour (normal/abnormal).
4. Intelligence (quite intelligent/not intelligent).
5. Memory (• short-term, • rescent, • long-term) good memory/amnesia.
6. Hallucinations (+/-), delusions (+/-).
7. Speech normal/abnormal = (Mutism, aphonia, dysarthria, dysphasia).

CRANIAL NERVES EXAMINATION

- CN I = Olfactory nerve = sensory
  Test: Sense of smell in each nostril
- CN II = Optic nerve = sensory
  Tests: (i) Acuity of vision = Snellen's method
       (ii) Field of vision = Perimetry
       (iii) Colour visioin = Ischiahara charts
- CN III, IV, VI = Oculomotor, trochlear and abducent nerves = motor
  Test = (i) Ocular movements
       (ii) Size of pupil and shape and mobility of pupil
- CN VII = Facial nerve = mixed
  Test:
  (i)   For sensory part = taste sensations over ant 2/3rd of tongue
  (ii) For motor parts = raising eyebrows, eye closure, blowing air, showing teeth
- CN V = Trigeminal nerve = mixed
  (i)   Test for sensory part = sensations over face, corneal reflex
  (ii) For motor part = messeters, pterygoids, and temporalis muscles action.
- CN VIII—auditory nerve = sensory
  Tests • Hearing • Rinne's test • Weber's test.
- CN IX, X = Glossopharyngeal and vagus nerves = mixed
  Tests: (i) Position of uvula (ii) Gag reflex.

- CN XI = Accessory nerve = motor.
  Test: Sternocleidomastoid and trapezium muscle actions.
- CN XII = Hypoglossal nerve = motor.
  Test: Movements of tongue.

MOTOR SYSTEM EXAMINATION

1. Bulk of muscle = Normal/atrophy/hypertrophy, equal/unequal on both sides.
2. Tone of muscle = Normal/hypotonia/hypertonia.
3. Power/strength of muscle= grades
   - 0 = Complete paralysis
   - 1 = Flicker of contraction
   - 2 = Movement but not against gravity
   - 3 = Movement present against gravity
   - 4 = Movement against resistance
   - 5 = Normal power.
4. Reflexes = (+/-) Grades
   - 0 = Absent
   - 1 = Present
   - 2 = Brisk
   - 3 = Very brisk
   - 4 = Clonus.
   (a) Superficial reflexes
   - Corneal reflexes (afferent = Vth CN), (efferent = VIIth CN)
   - Abdominal reflex (T_7 to T_{12})
   - Cremesteric reflex ($L_{1,2}$)
   - Planter reflex ($L_5 S_1$).
   (b) Deep tendon reflex
   - Biceps (C5,6)
   - Triceps (C6,7)
   - Supinator (C5,6)
   - Knee (L2,3,4)
   - Ankle (S1,2).
5. Coordination (i) finger nose test, (ii) walking in straight line, (iii) heel knee test.
6. Involuntary movements = tremers, chorea, dystonia, myoclonus, fasciculations, etc.
7. Gait = Normal/abnormal (specify).

SENSORY SYSTEM EXAMINATION

A. Superficial sensations (+/–)
- Touch
- Pain (superficial and deep)
- Temperature.
B. Deep sensitive (+/–)
- Position sense
- Vibration sense.
C. Discriminative sensory function (normal/abnormal)
- Astereognosis
- Two-point discriminative function
- Localization of touch.

5. HISTORY TAKING IN PEDIATRICS

INFORMANT: VERY IMPORTANT, CLOSE FAMILY MEMBER.

MOTHER IS PREFERRED (FATHER IS NOT PREFERRED)

1. *Personal:* Name, age, sex, address.
2. *Presenting complaint in chronological order*
   - Hospitalization should be separated out.
3. *History of present illness*
   - Illness progression
   - History of Rx taken
   - Recurrent history.
4. *Past history*
   - Number of similar illness in past (eventful)
   - Illness of common infection
   - Severe illness.
5. *Family history*
   a. Economical and social = complete social background
      - Living circumstances
      - Parenteral occupation and education
      - Income.
   b. Medical
      - Similar disease in family (present and past)
      - Severe disease
      - Infectious disease like TB, etc.

ANTENATAL, GROWTH DEVELOPMENT, NUTRITION AND IMMUNIZATION HISTORY

NUTRITION: ADEQUACY OF DIET COMPONENTS IS IMPORTANT.

Components (i) Present diet, (ii) Premorbid diet.

(a) *Present diet:* has the illness affected the dietary intake? (qualitative or quantitative)

Child < 3 years = diet determine by mother = Infant,
   - Other influences on mother
   - Infant feeding practices.

(b) *Premorbid diet:* Normal diet of child
   i. Breastfeeding
      - Initiation

- Prelacteal feeds
- Frequency (by clock or by demand)
- Total duration of feeding
- Difficulty in feeding, etc (from one or both breasts).

ii. *Top milk feeding:* whether gives or not
   - If given what is the milk given
   - Powder, goat, DMS, mother dairy, buffallo, cow, etc).
   - How diluted (Baby require full cream milk)
   - Mode of feeding, spoon or nipple, hygiene is important
     - Bottle and nipple hygiene is important
     - Keep bottle and nipple in boiling water (15 min) after every use and should not be touched before use
     - Mother's personal hygiene is important
   - Age at which it initiated
   - Total amount given is important.

iii. History of weaning
   - Semisolids and solids, etc, age of starting
   - Amount of starting
   - Child's acceptance.

IMMUNOLOGICAL HISTORY

- If immunization done accordingly or not
  Indicates: Route of diagnosis.
  adv: Child health advise + prevention advise.

DEVELOPMENTAL HISTORY

- Developmental peculiarities
  Normal development of muscles = cephalocaudal direction
- Abnormal growth, etc. diagnosis
- Developmental milestones
  1. *Social smile:* response to social response = 6-8 weeks
     Abnormal = beyond 10th week.
  2. *Head control:* moving head in all directions
     Normal = 3-4 months up to 6th months
     Abnormal beyond 6 months.
  3. *Rolling over:* rolls in bead supine to prone
     Normal = 5-6 months upto 7th month, abnormal beyond 7th month.

4. *Sitting*
   a. With support = Normal 6th month
   b. Without support = Normal 7-8th month.
5. *Crawling on limbs:* Normal 9-10 months.
6. *Standing*
   a. With support = Normal 10-11th month
   b. Without support = Normal 12-18 month Abnormal if > 18th month.

- *Birth history:* Place, gestation, direction of labour, type of delivery, Abnormal symptom in 1st week of life.
- *Antenatal history:* Drugs, radiation, etc in 1st trimester abortions, etc.

6. GENERAL PHYSICAL EXAMINATION IN PEDIATRICS

Sequence: (i) Vitals, (ii) Anthropometry, (GPE).

VITALS

(1) *Temperature:* Recorded at axilla, groin or rectum (rectal thermometer).

(2) *Pulse:* 1-6 yrs = HR is counted
Normal 80-130.

(3) *Size of cuff* = 3 × 8 cm or 5 × 12 cm
For ideal size the length should cover 2/3rd of arm.
Flush method: systolic BP can be measured. Sometimes pseudohypertension is recorded due to abnormal size of cuff.

(4) *Respiratory rate:* Normal 30-50/min, adult = 14-18/min.

ANTHROPOMETRY

Normal growth and development of child
- Head circumference
- Midarm circumference
- Chest circumference
- Height/length (< 2 yrs of age)
- Weight (gm).

GENERAL PHYSICAL EXAMINATION

Cries (i) Normal = well sustained.
(ii) Sick = poorly sustained.
(iii) Respiratory disorder = forced cry.

CRY INDICATES THE CONDITION OF CHILD.

EXAMINATION

1. *Face*
   - Epicanthic folds
   - Low set ears if 1/3rd of pinna is not upto line horizontal draw from lateral epicanthus
   - Mongolism, etc.
   - Cleft palate/cleft lip/both.
2. *Head*
   - Size, circumference

- Abnormal findings
- Fontenella normally is one ant and one post = presented at birth

  Anl diamond shaped = upto 18th months = at the level of head if raised indicated raised into cranial pressure due to any reason.

  If depressed shows any dehydration, etc.

  Post: Close at 8-9 months diamond shaped if do not close at right time, e.g. in rickets.
- Shape of skull: may be abnormal, e.g. in Caput quadratum, Cephalhematoma, etc.

3. *Hair*
   - Colour: black, brownish, whitish (malnutrition)
   - Quality also indicates malnutrition
   - Any fungal injection.

4. *Eyes*
   - Colour of sclera—abnormal is brownish
   - Conjunctival examination = pallor, etc.
   - Nystagmus, dehydration, glaucoma, etc.
   - Eyes are sunken in dehydration.

5. *Ear*
   - Abnormal formation
   - Hearing tests.

6. *Neck*
   - Cystic hygroma
   - Congenital cyanosis (may be central or peripheral)
   - Fistulas (Brachial fistulas)
   - Any abnormal findings.

7. *Hands*
   - Clubbing (may be due to cirrhosis of liver, hypoxia subacute myocarditis)
   - Grading of clubbing grade I, II, III, IV
   - Palmer edema, etc.
   - Any another abnormal finding.

8. *Lower limbs*
   - Any edema
   - Capillary filling time normal = < 3 sec
   - If > 3 sec indicates anemia, shock, etc.
   - While recording capillary filling time limbs should not be cold.

NOTE

1. **SIGNS OF DEHYDRATION**
   - Depression of ant fontenelles
   - Loss of skin moisture
   - Sunken eyes
   - Severe dehydration → shock.

2. **SIGNS OF SHOCK**
   - ↑ in capillary filling time > 3 sec
   - Decrease in urine quantity
   - Tachycardia
   - ↓ BP.

SYSTEMIC EXAMINATION

Same as medicine.

Note:

N^m	=	Normal
Ab^n	=	Abnormal
↑	=	Increase
↓	=	Decrease.

7. SURGERY PROFORMA FOR CASE PRESENTATION

BREAST

A. HISTORY

1. *Age and social status*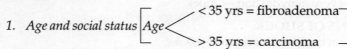

2. *History of lump*
   - Duration
   - Mode of onset
   - Progression
   - Pain
   - Associated symptoms (Fever, retraction of nipple, etc)
   - Presence of other lumps

3. *History of anorexia:* History of weight loss, history of bone pain, history of cough hemoptysis

4. *Discharge*
   - Absent
   - Present = colour, amount, blood, any foul smell.

5. *History of past illness*
   ⇨ TB
   ⇨ DM
   ⇨ Ht disease
   ⇨ HT
   ⇨ Similar problem

6. *Personal history*
   ⇨ Menstrual history
   ⇨ Marital status (Age of marriage)
   ⇨ Age at birth of first child, breastfeeding
   ⇨ History of oral contraceptives
   ⇨ Diet, addictions

7. *Family history*
   ⇨ Any similar complaint
   ⇨ TB
   ⇨ DM → Ht disease

B. EXAMINATION

Includes the following
1. General physical examination
2. Local examination
3. Systemic examination

1. GENERAL PHYSICAL EXAMINATION
   (see page 206)

2. LOCAL EXAMINATION

POSITION OF PATIENT

1. Sitting posture
2. Semirecumbent (45°) position
3. Recumbent position
4. Bending forward position
→ Most of examination is done in sitting posture
→ Semirecumbent position is ideal.

INSPECTION: INSPECTION IS DONE WITH

1. Arms on side of the body
2. Arms raised above head
3. Hands on hip
4. Bending forward

1. *Breast:* Compare both the breasts
   a. Position
   b. Size and shape
   c. Any puckering/dimpling
   d. Different in level
   e. Symmetry
2. *Skin over breast:* Note the following:
   a. Colour and texture
   b. Engorged veins
   c. Dimpling retraction, puckering
   d. Peau d' orange appearance
   e. Nodules, swelling
   f. Ulceration, fungation

3. *Nipple and areola*
   a. Presence and number
   b. Position
      - Compare level from other site
      - Vertical distance from clavicle
      - Horizontal distance from midline
   c. Surface, discharge
   d. Areola = colour, size, surface and texture
4. Arm and thorax
5. Axilla and supraclavicular fossa
   Must be inspected
   (Note: Inspection should be done in all positions).

PALPATION

- Palpation is done in sitting position ⇒ Semirecumbent position ⇒ recumbent position
- Palpate with the flat of fingers and the normal breast first
- Palpate all four quadrants and nipple
- Lump
  1. Local temperature and tenderness
  2. Site and number
  3. Size and shape
  4. • Surface, margin ⟨ Smooth = benign swelling
                       Rough = carcinoma
     • Margin ⟨ Regular
               Irregular
     • Consistency ⟨ firm, rubber = fibroadenosis
                    stony hard = carcinoma
  5. Fluctuation and transillumination (do not comment if tumor is hard)
  6. Fixity to
     ⇨ Skin
     ⇨ Breast tissue
     ⇨ Underlying fascia and muscles
     ⇨ Chest wall
- Examination of lymph nodes (Palpation)
  a. Axillary
     ⇨ Anterior (Pectoral)
     ⇨ Posterior (Subscapularis)

⇨ Lateral (Brachial)
⇨ Control
⇨ Optical
b. Supraclavicular
c. Deep cervical

(Note: If there is any ulcer examine like ulcer).

3. SYTEMIC EXAMINATION

Examine the following
1. Liver
2. Abdomen for lump, free fluid
3. Lungs
4. Bones—spine and long bones
5. PV and PR (Krukenberg's tumor).

PROSTATE

HISTORY

⇨ Describe each symptom
⇨ Symptoms of prostatism are
   i. Irritative symptom
      ⇨ Nocturia
      ⇨ Frequency
      ⇨ Urgency
      ⇨ Urge incontinence
      ⇨ Nocturnal incontinence (Enuresis)
   ii. Obstructive symptoms
      ⇨ Hesitancy
      ⇨ Poor flow (not improved by straining)
      ⇨ Dribbling
      ⇨ Intermittent stream
      ⇨ Sensation of poor bladder emptying
      ⇨ Retention (Acute/chronic)
⇨ History of UTI, history of trauma
⇨ History of calculi (pain)
⇨ History of discharge
⇨ History of contact (Infection)
⇨ History of instrumentation, stricture formation
⇨ History of any lymp (Hydronephrosis)
⇨ History of anorexia, weight loss, back pain, ⎤ Malignancy+
   limitation of movement, hemoptysis,   ⎥ metastasis
   bone pain   ⎦
⇨ History of acute retention (no passage of urine, suprapubic pain)

EXAMINATION

Examination includes (i) GPE, (ii) Local examination, (iii) Systemic examination

1. **GENERAL PHYSICAL EXAMINATION =**
   Same (see page 206)

2. **LOCAL EXAMINATION=** (I) DRE (II) SPINE
   TENDERNESS
   (i) DRE (digital rectal examination) = PR

POSITION OF PATIENT

   (i)   left lateral position = Sim's position = most popular position
   (ii) Dorsal position = on his back = in too ill-patients
   (iii) The knee elbow position
   (iv) Right lateral position
   (v)   Lithotomy position

⇨ Grading of BHP:
   Grade I: Can get above swelling easily
   Grade II: Can get above swelling with difficulty
   Grade III: Cannot get above swelling

⇨ Note the following about swelling
   i.   Size (approx)
   ii.   Surface, margin and consistency
   iii. Any nodularity
   iv.   Median sulcus
   v.   Elasticity
   vi.   Overlying rectal mucus (Fixed/not fixed)
   vii. Any discharge after PR

• Consistency, elasticity and nodularity indicate carcinoma.
• Normal prostate: palpable anteriorly = firm, rubbery, bilobed
  smooth surface, shallow central sulcus and rectal mucosa can
  be freely moved over it.
• Structures felt on DRE (normally)
  Anteriorly:
  • Prostate, seminal vesicle, base of bladder, rectovaginal pouch
    of peritoneum
  • Uterus, cervix, vagina, pouch of Douglas
  Laterally:
  • Ischiorectal fossa, lateral wall of pelvis, lower end of uterus,
    internal iliac arteries
  • Fallopian tubes, ovaries
  Posteriorly:
  • Hollow of sacrum, coccyx

⇨ Bull horn sign = Tenderness on deep press and discharge on PR

3. SYSTEMIC EXAMINATION

Examine abdomen, spine for metastatic evidences

OBS JAUNDICE

HISTORY

➡ Age (carcinoma in old patient, congenital in child, 40-50 years = gallstones) for cause

➡ History of weight loss and anorexia (hepatitis + malignancy)

➡ History of altered bowel habit and history of rashes

➡ History of pain in abdomen with radiation to back

➡ History of abdominal crisis and history of pruritis (describe)

➡ History of surgery (of abdomen or in childhood) (suggests choledochal cyst/stricture)

➡ History of intolerance to fatty food (Indicates gallbladder disease)

➡ History of colicky pain in abdomen, dark coloured urine

➡ History of flatulence dyspepsia

➡ History of drugs
  - Hepatotoxic drugs
    - Antitubercular drugs
    - Halothane
    - Valproic acid and others
  - Associated with gallstones
    - Clofibrate
    - Cholestyramine
    - Oral contraceptive pills
  - Others
    - Phenothiazine (Cholestatic jaundice)

➡ Other lumps and past history
  H/o DM= carcinoma of pancreas (Common)
  H/o TB = LN enlargement and TB of liver

EXAMINATION

(1) GPE (2) Abdominal examination

i. GENERAL PHYSICAL EXAMINATION (SEE PAGE 206)

➡ *Pulse* i. Bradycardia (bile on SA node)
  ii. Bounding pulse (Liver cell failure)

➡ Temperature = Increased in cholangiitis and hepatitis

➡ Scratch marks, nails shiny, icterus, signs of malnutrition

➡ Signs of liver cell failure

ii. ABDOMINAL EXAMINATION
  ⇨ Distension (If present may be due to ascites)
  ⇨ Liver
    ⇨ Almost always enlarged in jaundice
    ⇨ Obstruction = firm, (If cholangiitis) and tender
    ⇨ Parenchymal = soft and tender
    ⇨ Metastatic = nodular
  ⇨ Spleen = enlarged (If PHT and hemolysis)
  ⇨ Gallbladder may be enlarged (due to carcinoma of pancreas, cholangiocarcinoma, ampullary or periampullary carcinoma, stricture)
  ⇨ On examination (Normal gallbladder)
    • Pyriform
    • Smooth
    • Continuous with liver
    • Moves with respiration
    • Cannot reach above it
  ⇨ Look for Murphy's sign and boas sign
  ⇨ Others = PR examination, chest examination, spine examination.

DIAGNOSIS
  ⇨ Prov diagnosis = Jaundice (Type: obstructive jaundice or nonobstructive jaundice)
    ⇨ If obs jaundice → site of obstruction (intra/extrahepatic)
    ⇨ Cause of obstruction (carcinoma/stones, etc).

PERIPHERAL VASCULAR DISEASES

HISTORY

1. *Intermittent claudication* (severe pain in calf muscles during walking but subsides with rest. Due to ischemia of nerves. Due to accummulation of P substance. Due to inadequate blood supply).

   Boyd's classification

   Grades

   Grade 1: Patient continue to walk and pain disappear.

   Grade 2: Patient has to walk with effort.

   Grade 3: Patient has to take rest.

   Grade 4: Rest pain.

2. *Rest pain:*
3. Gangrene
4. Superficial thrombophlebitis (pain, redness, swelling, fever → Buerger's disease)
5. History of pain in upper limbs in writing and lifting weight.
6. History of paresthesia (Numbness, tingling sensation).
7. History of impotence.
8. Others:
   - History of joint pain
   - Swelling in ankle (Deep vein thrombosis)
   - Back pain (Disc prolapse)
   - Chest pain, dyspnoea (Embolism)
   - Fainting, blackouts, blurring of vision (General athero-sclerosis)
   - History of local trauma.

NOTE: SIGNS OF GANGRENE
- Changing colour
- Decrease in temperature
- Loss of sensation, palsation, function.

GENERAL PHYSICAL EXAMINATION (SEE PAGE 206)

LOCAL EXAMINATION

INSPECTION

1. Changing colour and signs of ischemia

2. Buerger's postural test
3. Capillary filling time (Nomal: 20-30 sec)
4. Venous refilling
5. Gangrene (Type and line of demarcation)

PALPATION

1. Skin temperature
2. Capillary refilling (Tip of nail) (Normal is few seconds)
3. Venous refilling
4. Crossed leg test
5. Cold and warm test [→ ice cold water (white) → warm water (blue) (due to cyanosis)]
6. Allen's test (For radial and ulnar arteries)
7. Palpation of gangrenous area (note the crepitations)
8. Palpation of big vessels:
   - Dorsalis pedis artery
   - Posterior tibial artery
   - Anterior tibial artery
   - Popliteal artery
   - Femoral artery
   - Radial and ulnar arteries
   - Subclavian artery
   - Common carotid artery
   - Superficial temporal artery
9. Examination of lymph nodes

DIFFERENTIAL DIAGNOSIS

- Buerger's disease
- Raynaud's disease
- Collagen vascular disease
- Atherosclerosis
- Embolic diseases
- Diabetes mellitus

THYROID

AIM

1. Whether thyroid palpable or not
2. Solitary or multiple nodule
3. Diffuse enlargement
4. Euthyroid
5. Retrosternal extension
6. Benign or malignant
7. Pressure effects

HISTORY

1. AGE

⇨ Simple/diffuse, hyperplastic = teenage, puberty and prepuberty

⇨ Colloid goitre/solitary and multinodular goitre = 20-30 years of age

⇨ Follicular = middle age woman

⇨ Hashimoto's disease = middle age woman

⇨ Papillary carcinoma = young girl

2. SEX

⇨ Majority in females: thyrotoxicosis = 8:1
                      thyroid carcinoma = 3:1

3. SWELLING

• Onset, duration, rate of growth, associated with pain or not (pain is due to haemorrhage in goitre, late stages of malignancy or inflammatory condition).

4. THYROID STATUS

• **Hypothyroidism**
  • Tiredness
  • Mental lethargy
  • Cold intolerance
  • Weight gain inspite poor appetite
  • Loss of hair (lateral 2/3rd of eyebrows)
  • Puffiness of face
  • Dry skin (decrease sweating)

- **Primary Hyperthyroidism**
  - Sleepness nights
  - Weight loss in spite of good appetite
  - Heat intolerance
  - Preference for cold
  - Excess sweating
  - Tremor of hand
  - Weakness of proximal muscles
  - Irritability
  - Protruding eyes (Diploplegia, ophthalmoplegia)
- **Secondary Thyrotoxicosis (CVS involvement is frequent)**
  - Palpitation
  - Precordial chest pain
  - Dyspnoea on exertion
  - Pedal edema
  - Orthopnoea
  - PND
  - No tremor or eye signs

5. PRESSURE EFFECTS

- Dysphagia/stridor/cough
- Enlargement of neck veins or superficial veins in chest wall
- Dysphagia
- Hoarseness of voice

6. FAMILY HISTORY

- Autoimmune diseases

7. TREATMENT HISTORY

- Effects and duration of treatment
- History of irradiation
- Intake of antithyroid drugs

EXAMINATION

GENERAL PHYSICAL EXAMINATION (SEE PAGE 206)

- Facies
  - Anxious, tense, irritable, exophthalmos = thyrotoxicosis
  - Loss of hair, mask like faces with no expression = hypothyroidism.
- Nails: Plummer's nail (Separation of finger nail from the nailbed, seen in thyrotoxicosis)

SIGNS OF HYPOTHYROIDISM

- Slow pulse rate
- Dry skin
- Cold extremities
- Periorbital puffiness
- Hoarse voice
- Bradykinesis
- Hung up ankle jerks

SIGNS OF MYXOEDEMA

- Fat accumulation at nape of neck and shoulder
- Supraclavicular puffiness
- Blotted lips with penting lips
- Yellow hinge to skin
- Voice is like gramophone record

SIGNS OF PRIMARY HYPERTHYROIDISM

- Sleeping tachycardia
  - Mild: Less than 90/minute
  - Moderate: 90-110/minute
  - Severe: More than 110/minute
- Moist skin
- Tremor in protruded tongue/outstreched hand
- Muscle weakness
- Pretibial myxoedema (shined plaque of thickness, skin with coarse hair which may be cyanotic when cold). In severe cases whole leg below knee is affected with clubbing of fingers and toes.
- Eye changes (lid retraction, exophthalmos, ophthalmoplegia, chemosis)

LOCAL EXAMINATION

1. INSPECTION

Pizillo's method → It is used to render inspection easier, i.e. hands are placed behind the neck and the patient is asked to push the head backwards against the clasped hand on the occiput.

NOTE THE FOLLOWING:

1. Site, size, extent, shape and edge of the swelling
2. Number of swellings, colour and overlying skin

3. Movement with deglutition
4. Prominent veins on the anterior part of thorax
5. Effect of protrusion of tongue
⇨ Thyroid moves up with deglutition
Others:
1. Thyroglossal cyst (with tongue protruding)
2. Subhyoid bursa
3. Pretracheal lymph nodes (fixed to trachea)
4. Prelaryngeal lymph nodes (fixed to larynx)
⇨ Lower border of swelling cannot be seen to move on deglutition in case of retrosternal goitre
⇨ Pemberton's sign: congestion of face and distress on rising both the arms over head until they touch the ear. Seen in retrosternal goitre due to obstruction of the thorasic inlet.
⇨ Causes of diffuse enlargement
- Physiological goitre
- Colloid goitre
- Graves' disease
- Hashimoto's disease

PALPATION

Palpation from behind with neck slightly flexed. Additional information about one lobe may be obtained by relaxing sternocleido-mastoid muscle of that side by fixing and rotating the face to the same side.

⇨ *Lahey's method:* Palpation of each lobe. In this, examiner stands in front of patient. To palpate the left lobe properly, the thyroid is pushed to left side from the right side by the left hand of the examiner.
⇨ *Crile's method:* Palpation using thumb placed on thyroid while patient is swallowing.

NOTE:

1. Temperature and tenderness.
2. Size, shape and extent, get below the thyroid gland
3. Edge, surface (smooth in primary thyrotoxicosis, bosselated in multinodular goitre), consistency (soft in colloid goitre, hard in Graves' disease and Hashimoto's disease)
4. Fluctuation, transillumination
5. Mobility (fixed in malignancy and chronic thyroiditis)

6. Impulse on coughing (plunger goitre). Whole of enlarge thyroid lie in superior mediastinum, no gland felt in neck, but goitre is seen when intrathorasic presssure rises during coughing.
7. Pressure effects:
   - Kocher's test: slight pressure on the lobes produces stridor if pressure is being exerted on trachea.
   - Horner's syndrome: exophthalmos, ptosis, myosis, loss of ciliospinal reflex.
   - Tracheal deviation
   - Berri's sign: enlarged gland displaces the carotid backwards and outwards so that it cannot be palpated in its normal position. It is then felt behind the posterior edge of swelling (in malignancy the carotid tends to be surrounded by tumor).
8. Cervical lymph nodes (enlarged/not enlarged)
9. Measurement of neck (circumference at the most prominent part of the swelling)

PERCUSSION

On manubrium sterni for retrosternal extension or mediastinal metastasis.

AUSCULTATION

Systolic bruit may be heard at the superior pole due to increase in vascularity.

8. PROFORMA FOR OBSTETRICS PRACTICAL CASE PRESENTATION

HISTORY

1. VITAL STATISTICS
- Name
- Age
- Occupation and religion
- Date of first examination
- Duration of marriage
- Gravida and parity (GPAL)
- Period of gestation = LMP and EDD, etc.

2. COMPLAINTS
- In chronological order with duration and mode of onset, progress and duration
- If no complaints then enquire about sleep, appetite, bowel habits, urination

3. HISTORY OF PRESENT PREGNANCY

T_1
- Nausea, vomiting
- Confirm the pregnancy
- Booked/unbooked
- No of visits to ANC
- Any lung exposure
- History of fever with rashes
- LPV, BPV
- Frequency of micturition, burning sensation
- Breast tenderness and fatigue

T_2
- Quickening
- TT immunization
- Dietary supplements
- LPV, BPV
- Dai interference
- History of PIH
  [Headache, wt gain, oligurea, pedel edema, epigastric pain, blurring of vision]

T_3
- Anaemia and heart disease
- PIH

- LPV, BPV
- Fe and FA intake
- History of blood transfusion

4. **OBSTETRICS HISTORY**
   - No of living children
   - For every child
     1. Date of birth
     2. Pregnancy and labour events
     3. Method of delivery
     4. Puerperium
     5. Baby
        - Weight and sex
        - Condition at birth
        - Duration of breastfed
        - Immunization
        - Present health status

5. **PAST HISTORY**
   - HT
   - DM
   - TB
   - Genetically transmitted disease
   - Surgical history

6. **HISTORY OF ALLERGY AND DRUG HISTORY**

7. **PERSONAL HISTORY**
   - Menstrual history (Cycle, duration, amount of flow, LMP)
   - Contraception
   - Food and bowel habits
   - Addictions (Smoking, alcohol, etc).

8. **FAMILY HISTORY**
   - HT
   - DM
   - TB
   - Genetically transmitted disease
   - Any relevant information.

EXAMINATION

1. **GENERAL PHYSICAL EXAMINATION (SEE PAGE 206)**
   - Height and weight
   - Tongue, teeth, gums tonsils
   - Rest is same

2. **BREAST EXAMINATION**
   - To note presence of pregnancy
   - To rule out any pathology
   - To note nipples and skin condition of areola
     [Purpose: To correct abnormality, if any, so that there will be no difficulty in breastfeeding immediately following delivery]

3. **CVS AND RESPIRATORY SYSTEM EXAMINATION**
   - To rule out any pathology

4. **ABDOMINAL EXAMINATION (WITH EMPTY BLADDER)**
   INSPECTION
   1. Skin condition
   2. Shape of uterus
   3. Contour of uterus
   4. Incisional scar mark, etc

   PALPATION
   1. Height of uterus (in weeks)
   2. Abdominal girth
   3. Obstetric grips
      1. Fundal grip
      2. Lateral/umbilical grip
      3. First pelvic grip
      4. Second pelvic grip

   AUSCULTATION
   1. FHS (Fetal heart sounds)
   2. Any abnormal sounds

5. **PV EXAMINATION (WITH EMPTY BLADDER)**
   INSPECTION
   1. Character of discharge, if any
   2. Any abnormal finding

   SPECULUM EXAMINATION
   1. Characteristic bluish red colouration of cervix in pregnancy
   2. Discharge, etc. from cervical os.
   3. Cervical smear for cytology.

   BIMANUAL EXAMINATION
   1. Uterus = size, shape, position, consistancy
   2. Cervix = consistancy direction, pathology
   3. Adnexae
      [Inference: (1) Lie, (2) Presentation, (3) Attitude, (4) Presenting part (5) Position].

APPENDIX 4

INVESTIGATIONS WITH NORMAL VALUES

1. **Hemoglobin (Hb)**
   - At birth = 23 gm%
   - Adults (M) = 14-18 gm%
   - Adults (F) = 12-16 gm%
   - Clinically (irrespective of sex) = 15 gm%

2. **Red Blood Cell Count (RBC)**
   - Male = 4.5 to 6.0 million / cu. mm
   - Female = 4.2 to 5.4 million / cu. mm.
   - Children = 6 to 7 million / cu. mm.
   - Clinically (irrespective of sex) = 5 million/mm^3
   - Reticulocyte count = 0.5 - 2.0% (average < 1%)

3. **White Blood Cell Count (WBC) or (TLC)**
   - Ranges from 4,000 - 11,000/ cu. mm. (adults)
   - 20,000/cu mm (at birth)

4. **DLC (Differential Leucocyte Count)**

	Adult	*Children*
a. Neutrophils	50-70%	20-30%
b. Lymphocytes	20-30%	50-70%
c. Monocytes	2-8%	2-7%
d. Basophils	0-2%	0-2%
e. Eosinophils	1-3%	1-4%.

5. **Absolute Eosinophil Count** = 40 - 440 cells/cu. mm.

6. **Packed cell volume (PCV)**
   - Male = 40- 50 %
   - Female = 38- 45 %
   - Mean corpuscular hemoglobin **(MCH)** = 27-31 pg
   - Mean corpuscular hemoglobin concentration **(MCHC)** = 32-36%
   - Mean corpuscular volume **(MCV)** = 76-96 cu. mm.

7. **Erythrocyte sedimentation rate (ESR)**
   - Male = 0-10 mm 1st hour (Wintrobe's Method)
   - Female = 0-20 mm 1st hour (Wintrobe's Method)

8. **Platelet count** = 1.5-4.5 lakhs/cu. mm.

9. **Coagulation**
   - Bleeding time = 2 - 6 minutes
   - Clotting time = 3 - 9 minutes
   - Prothrombin time = 12-16 s

10. **Blood pH** = 7.35-7.45 (venous - artery)
    (**pH**- hydrogen ion concentration which helps in denoting acidity or alkalinity of the solution (variation from 1- 14, i.e. from most acid to most alkali)

11. **Electrolytes**
    - Serum Sodium = 135 - 145 mEq/L
    - Serum Potassium = 3.5 - 5.5 mEq/L
    - Serum Chloride = 98 - 106 mEq/L
    - Serum Bicarbonate = 22 - 26 mEq/L
    - Serum Lithium = 0.2 - 1.0 mEq/L

12. **Serum Protein:**
    - Total = 6 - 8 gm%
    - Albumin = 3.5 - 5.5 gm
    - Globulins = 2 - 3 gm%
    - A/G ratio = 1.7:1
    - Fibrinogen = 0.3 mg%
    - Prothrombin = 40 mg%

13. **Total Serum Bilirubin:**
    - Total = 0.3 to 1.0 mg /dl
    - Direct Bilirubin = < 0.3 mg /dl
    - Indirect Bilirubin = < 0.8 mg /dl
    - **Serum Alkaline Phosphatase = 25 - 90.** U/L
    - **Serum Lactic Dehydrogenase = 60 - 320** U/L
    - **SGOT** or Alanine aminotransferase (ALT) = 5 - 40 U/L
    - **SGPT** or Aspartate aminotransferase (AST) = 5 - 35 U/L

14. **Blood Glucose**
    - Fasting = 70 - 110 Mg / dl
    - Post prandial (after food ,1 ¾ hours) =100 -140 mg / dl

15. **Kidney functions test**
    - Blood urea = 20 - 40 mg%
    - Serum creatinine = 0.6 - 1.2 mg%

16. **Serum Cholesterol = 150 - 240 mg / dl**

17. **Serum Creatinine** = 0.8 - 1.4 mg / dl

18. **Serum Uric Acid** = 3.0 - 7.0 mg / dl

19. **Serum Calcium** = 9.0 - 11.0 mg / dl

20. **Serum Phosphorus** = 3.5 - 5.5 Mg / dl

21. **Serum Amylase** = 25 - 90 U/L

22. **Serum Copper** = 70 - 150 mg / dl

23. **C-reactive Protein** = <10 mg/L

24. **Creatine Kinase (CPK)**
    - Male < 170 U/L
    - Female < 130 U/L

25. **Serum Iron** = 60 - 160 mg%

26. **Serum Ferritin**
    - Males = 15 - 300 µg/L
    - Females = 15 - 150 µg/L

27. **Blood Urea Nitrogen** = 10 - 20 mg%

28. **Serum Magnesium** = 1 - 2 mg%

29. **Serum Ceruloplasmin** = 200 - 300 µg/L

30. **Serum Phosphate** = 3.0 - 4.5 mg%

31. **Serum Gamma Glutamyl Transpeptidase**
    - Male = 11-50 U/L
    - Female = 07-32 U/L

32. **Immunoglobulins**
    - IgA = 0.8 - 4 g/L
    - IgG = 5.5 - 16.5 g/L
    - IgM = 0.4 - 2.0 g/L

33. **Prostate-specific Antigen (PSA)** = up to 4.0 µg/L

34. **Lipid Profile** should be done after 12 hours fasting
    - Total = 350 - 800 mg%
    - Triglycerides = 30 - 150 mg%
    - Phospholipids = 150 - 300 mg%
    - HDL = > 40 mg%
    - LDL = < 180 mg%

- VLDL = < 40 mg%
- FFA = 10 - 30 mg %
- Cholesterol = 150 - 250 mg% (free = 28%)

35. **Urine Normal Values**
    - Colour = Colourless
    - Reaction = Acidic
    - Specific gravity = 1.010 to 1.030
    - pH = 5.6 - 6.5
    - Sugar = Nil
    - Albumin = Nil
    - Ketone = Nil
    - Urobilinogen = 0.3 - 1.0 mg/dL
    - Bilirubin = Nil
    - Bile salt = Nil
    - Pus cells = Nil/HPF
    - RBCs = Nil/HPF
    - Epithelial cells = Nil/HPF
    - Casts, crystals = Nil/HPF
    - Calcium = 0 - 300 mg/24 hours
    - Protein = < 0.15 g/24 hours
    - pH = 5.0 - 8.0
    - Specific Gravity = 1.001 - 1.035
    - RBCs, WBCs, Pus cells should be Nil

36. **Sugar Test in Urine:** Should be done after 2 hours of food intake. Also collecting of mid-stream urine is important for accurate analysis. Presence of sugar is analyzed by two methods now, i.e. one by old benedict's reagents and another by latest dipsticks. In case of Benedict's test, if results shows
    - Blue colour = Nil
    - Green colour = + (0.1 - 0.5 g/dl)
    - Yellow colour = ++ (0.5 - 1.0 g/dl)
    - Orange colour = +++ (1.0 - 1.5 g/dl)
    - Brick red colour = ++++ (1.5 - 2.0 g/dl)

37. **Blood gases**

	Arterial	Venous
- pH	7.35-7.45	7.35-7.45
- PO$_2$	95-100 mmHg	40 mmHg
- PCO$_2$	35-40 mmHg	46 mmHg
- O$_2$ saturation	≥ 97%	—

38. **Semen Analysis**
    - Volume = 2.5-3.5 ml per ejaculation
    - Colour = White, opalescent
    - Specific gravity = 1.028
    - pH = 7.35 to 7.50
    - Sperm count = 80-120 million/ml (avg = 100 million/ml)
    - Motility = > 80% sperms with normal morphology

39. **Hormones** (serum levels)
    - Testosterone
      Males = 7000 μg/L (daily secretion = 7 mg)
      Females = 370 μg/L (daily secretion = 350 μg)
    - Growth hormone (plasma level) = 3 ng/ml
    - Plasma insulin level = 10-50 μU/ml
    - Serum progesterone
      Males = 0.3 ng/ml
      Females = 0.9 ng/ml, 18 ng/ml (during follicular phase)
    - Serum prolactin
      Males = 5 ng/ml
      Females = 8 ng/ml

40. **Thyroid function tests**
    - TSH = 10 pmol/L
    - T3
      Total = 3 μg%
      Free = 1.5 ng%
    - T4
      Total = 8 μg%
      Free = 2 ng%
    - TBP (thyroxine-binding globulin) = 1-2 ng%

41. **Blood culture**
    - Done for detection of infection and to find out the type of organism
    - Normal = No growth

42. **Urine culture**
    - Done for detection of UTI and to find out the organism
    - Normal = No growth

APPENDIX 5

SOME IMPORTANT DEFINITIONS

Achlorhydria: Absence of HCl in stomach.

Acidosis: A condition in which the acidity of body fluids and tissues is abnormally high.

Acquired means anything that is not present at birth but develops some time later. An acquired condition is new in the sense that it is not genetic (inherited) and added in the sense that was not present at birth.

Acromegaly: Increase in size of hands, feet, face due to excessive production of growth hormone by a tumor of the anterior pituitary gland.

Acute means of abrupt onset, in reference to a disease. Acute often also connotes an illness that is of short duration, rapidly progressive, and in need of urgent care.

Addison's disease: A syndrome due to inadequate secretion of corticosteroid hormones by adrenal glands.

Adenoma: A benign tumor of epithelial origin that is derived from glandular tissue.

Adverse effect: A harmful or abnormal result. An adverse effect may be caused by administration of a medication or by exposure to a chemical and be indicated by an untoward result such as by illness or death.

Adverse reaction: any unexpected or dangerous reaction to a drug. An unwanted effect caused by the administration of a drug. The onset of the adverse reaction may be sudden or develop over time.

Afebrile: Not showing any sign of fever (at Normal body temperature).

Ageusia is inability to taste sweet, sour, bitter, or salty substances. Some people can taste but their ability to do so is reduced, they are said to have hypogeusia.

Agglutination: Clumping = the sticking together.

Aging: The process of becoming older, a process that is genetically determined and environmentally modulated.

Alkalosis: A condition in which the alkalinity of body fluids and tissues is abnormally high.

Alzheimer's disease: A progressive neurological disease of the brain that leads to the irreversible loss of neurons and dementia.

Anaerobic: Not requiring oxygen. Anaerobic bacteria do not need oxygen to grow in fact, oxygen is usually toxic to them. An anaerobic environment lacks oxygen.

Analgesia: The inability to feel pain while still conscious.

Anemia: The condition of having less than the normal number of red blood cells or less than the normal quantity of hemoglobin in the blood or both. The oxygen-carrying capacity of the blood is, therefore, decreased.

Aneurysm: A localized widening (dilatation) of an artery, vein, or the heart. At the area of an aneurysm, there is typically a bulge and the wall is weakened and may rupture. The word aneurysm means a widening.

Angina is chest pain due to an inadequate supply of oxygen to the heart muscle. The chest pain of angina is typically severe and crushing. There is a feeling just behind the breastbone (the sternum) of pressure and suffocation.

Anorexia: Loss of appetite.

Anorexia nervosa: A psychological illness, most common in females adolescents, in which the patient has no desire to eat.

Antagonist: A drug or other substance with opposite action to that of another drug.

Antibiotic: A substance, produced or desired by a microorganism that destroys or inhibit the growth of the microorganisms.

Antibody: An immunoglobulin, a specialized immune protein, produced because of the introduction of an antigen into the body, and which possesses the remarkable ability to combine with the very antigen that triggered its production.

Anticoagulant: An agent that prevents the clotting of blood.

Anticoagulant: Any agent used to prevent the formation of blood clots.

Antigen: Any substance that the body regards as or potentially dangerous and against which it produce an antibody.

Antihistamine: A drug that inhibits some of the effects of histamine in the body, in particular its role in allergic condition.

Antispasmotic: A drug that relieves spasm of smooth muscle.

Anuria: Failure of kidneys to produce urine.

Anxiety: A feeling of apprehension, worry, uneasiness, or esp. of the future.

Aplasia: Total or partial failure of development of an organ or tissue.

Apoptosis: A form of cell death in which a programmed sequence of events leads to the elimination of cells without releasing harmful substances into the surrounding area. Apoptosis plays a crucial role in developing and maintaining health by eliminating old cells, unnecessary cells, and unhealthy cells. The human body replaces perhaps a million cells a second.

Arrhythmia: An abnormal heart rhythm. In an arrhythmia the heartbeats may be too slow, too rapid, too irregular, or too early. Rapid arrhythmias (greater than 100 beats per minute) are called tachycardias. Slow arrhythmias (slower than 60 beats per minute) are called bradycardias. Irregular heart rhythms are called fibrillations (as in atrial fibrillation and ventricular fibrillation). When a single heartbeat occurs earlier than normal, it is called a premature contraction.

Arthritis: Inflammation of one or more joints, characterised by swelling, warmth, redness of the underlying skin, pain and restriction of movement.

Asthma: A common disorder in which chronic inflammation of the bronchial tubes (bronchi) makes them swell, narrowing the airways. Asthma involves only the bronchial tubes and does not affect the air sacs (alveoli) or the lung tissue (the parenchyma of the lung) itself.

A disease caused by hyperresponsive of the tracheobronchial tree to various stimuli.

Atherosclerosis: A disease of arteries in which fatty plaques develop on their inner walls, with eventual obstruction of blood flow.

Autoimmunity: A condition characterised by a specific humoral or cell-mediated immune response against the constituents of the body's own tissues (auto antigens). It may result in hypersensitivity reaction or if severe, in autoimmune disease.

Bacteria: Single-celled microorganisms which can exist either as independent (free-living) organisms or as parasites (dependent upon another organism for life).

Basophil: Any structure, cell, or histologic element staining readily with basic dye.

Belching: Expulsion of gas from stomach with sound production.

Blanching: To loose colour.

Bradycardia: Slowness of heart beat as evidenced by slowing of the pulse rate < 60/min.

Cancer: Any malignant, cellular tumor, cancers are divided into two broad categories of carcinoma and sarcoma.

Carbuncle: A necrotising infection of skin and subcutaneous tissues composed of cluster of fruncles.

Carcinoma: A malignant new growth made up of epithelial cells tending to infiltrate surrounding tissues and to give rise to metastasis.

Cardiocentesis: Surgical puncture of the heart.

Cardiorrhexis: Rupture of heart.

Catabolism: Any destructive process, by which complex substances are converted by living cells into more simple compounds, with release of energy.

Chancroid: A nonsyphilitic veneral disease transmitted by direct contact, and caused by *Haemophilus ducreyi.*

Chronic: This important term in medicine comes from the Greek chronos, time and means lasting a long time.

Cirrhosis: Intestinal inflammation of an organ, particularly liver.

Clinical: Having to do with the examination and treatment of patients or applicable to patients.

Colic: Acute paroxysmal abdominal pain.

Colitis: Inflammation of colon.

Coma: A stage of profound unconsciousness from which the patient cannot be aroused even by powerful stimuli.

Conception: The onset of pregnancy.

Convulsion: An involuntary contraction or series of contractions of the voluntary muscles.

Coryza: Profuse discharge from mucous membrane of nose.

Cretinism: Arrested physical and mental development with dystrophy of bones and soft tissues, due to congenital lack of thyroid secretion.

Culture: The propagation of microorganisms or of living tissue cells in media conductive to their growth.

Cyanosis: A bluish discolouration of skin and mucous membranous due to excessive concentration of reduced hemoglobin in the blood.

Cyst: Any closed epithelium-lined cavity or sac, normal or abnormal, usually containing liquid or semisolid material.

Delirium: A mental disturbance of relatively short duration usually reflecting a toxic state, marked by illusions, hallucinations, delusions, excitement, restlessness and incoherence.

Delusion: A false personal belief based on incorrect inference about external reality and firmly maintained in spite of incontrovertible and obvious proof or evidence to the contrary.

Dementia: Organic loss of intellectual functions.

Dialysis: The process of separating crystalloids and colloids in solution by the difference in their rates of diffusion through readily colloids very slowly or not at all.

Diarrhea: Frequent passage of unformed watery bowel movements.

Diastole: The dilation, or the period of dilation.

Dizziness: Sensation of unsteadyness and feedling of movement instead.

Drowsiness: State of almost falling asleep.

Dystonia: Impairment of muscle tone.

Dysuria: Painful or difficult urination.

Eczema: A superficial inflammation of skin mainly affecting the epidermis.

Edema: Excessive accumulation of fluid in the body tissues.

Embolus: A clot or other plug brought by the blood from another vessel and forced into a smaller one thus obstructing the circulation.

Endoparasite: Parasite that lives inside its host, for example in liver, lungs, gut, or other tissues of the body.

Eosinophilia: An increase in the number of eosinophils in the blood.

Epistaxis: Haemorrhage from the nose.

Eructation: Producing gas from stomach, usually with a characteristic sound.

Eruption: The appearance of a lesion such as redness or spotting on the skin or mucous membrane.

Exogenous: Originating outside the body or part of the body.

Expectorant: A drug that enhances the secretion of sputum by the air passage so that it is easier to cough up.

Fainting: Temporary loss of consciousness due to decrease cerebral blood flow.

Fibrillation: A rapid and choatic beating of the many individual muscle fibres of the heart, which is consequently, unable to maintain effective synchronous contraction.

Fissure: A groove or cleft.

Flaccid: Flabby and lacking is firmness.

Flatulence: Excessive gas production in stomach and intestine.

Gastritis: Inflammation of the linking of stomach.

Gastroenteritis: Inflammation of the stomach and intestine.

Geriatrics: The branch of medicine concerned with the diagnosis and treatment of disorders that occur in old age.

Glossitis: Inflammation of tongue.

Gonorrhea: Veneral disease, caused by the bacterium, *Neisseria gonorrhoea*, that affects the genital mucous membrane of either sex.

Gout: A disease in which a defect in uric acid metabolism causes an excess of the uric acid and its slts to accumulate in the bloodstream and joints.

Gynaecomastia: Excessive development of the male mammary glands, even to functional state.

Hallucinations: A perception of something that is not really there.

Heartburn: Discomfort of pain usually burning in character, that is felt behind the breast bone and often appears to rise from the upper mid abdomen towards into the throat.

Hematuria: The presence of blood in urine.

Hemodialysis: A technique of removing waste materials or poisons from the blood using the principle or dialysis.

Hemostatic: An agent that stops or prevents hemorrhages.

Hepatitis: Inflammation of liver due to a virus infection or such diseases as amoebic dysentery and lupus.

Hepatomegaly: Enlargement of liver to such extent that it can be felt below the rib margin.

Hirsutism: Abnormal coarse and excessive hairness, especially in women or exceptive hair growth.

Hyperesthesia: Excessive sensibility (nerves) especially of skin.

Hyperglycemia: Low blood glucose level (below normal level).

Hyperkalemic: Excessive K^+ in blood.

Hyperlipoproteinemia: An excess of lipoproteins in blood due to a disorder of lipoprotein metabolism.

Hypernatremia: Excess of Na^+ in blood.

Hyperparathyroidism: Excessive activity of the parathyroid glands.

Hyperplasia: A condition in which there is an increase in the number of normal cells in a tissue or organ.

Hyperplasia: Abnormal increase in the number of normal cells, in Nm awareness in an organ or tissue which increases its volume.

Hypersensitivity: A state of altered reactivity in which the body reacts with an exaggerated immune response to a foreign body.

Hypertension: Persistently high blood pressure (above normal value).

Hypertrophy: Enlargement or overgrowth of an organ or part of the body due to the increased size of the constituent cells.

Hyperuricemia: Excessive uric acid in blood.

Hypokalemia: Low K^+ in blood.

Hypoplasia: Incomplete development or underdevelopment of an organ/tissue.

Hypotension: Abnormally low blood pressure.

Hypovolemia: Abnormally * volume circulating fluids (plasma) in the body.

Hypoxia: Reduction of blood supply to a tissue below physiological levels despite adequate perfusion of the tissue by blood.

Hysteria: A neurosis with symptoms based on conversion, characterised by lack of control over acts and emotions.

Iatrogenic: Resulting from the activity of physicians.

Idiopathic: Occurring without known cause.

Ileus: Intestinal obstruction.

Immunodeficiency: A deficiency of the immune response due to hypoactivity or numbers of lymphoid cells.

Immunosuppression: The artificial prevention of the immune response as by use of radiation antimetabolites.

In situ: In the normal location. An *"in situ"* tumor is one that is confined to its site of origin and has not invaded neighboring tissue or gone elsewhere in the body.

In vitro: Literally in glass, as in a test tube. A test that is performed *in vitro* is one that is done in glass or plastic vessels in the laboratory.

In vivo: In the living organism, as opposed to *in vitro* (in the laboratory).

Infarct: A localised area of ischemic necrosis produced by occlusion of the arterial supply of the venous drainage of the part.

Inflammation: A basic way in which the body reacts to infection, irritation or other injury, the key feature being redness, warmth, swelling and pain. Inflammation is now recognized as a type of nonspecific immune response.

Inflammation: A protective tissue response to injury or destruction of tissues, which serves to destroy, dilute or wash off both the injurious agent and the injured tissues.

Irritable bowel syndrome: A chronic noninflammatory disease with a psychophysiologic basis, characterised by abdominal pain, diarrhoea, or constipation or both, and no detectable pathologic change; a variant form is marked by painless diarrhoea.

* = Low

Ischemia: Blood supply is a part, due to functional constriction or actual obstruction of a blood vessel.

Jaundice: Condition characterised by yellowness of skin, sclera of eyes, mucous membranous and body fluids due to deposition of bile pigment resulting from excess bilirubin in the blood.

Ketosis: Accumulation of excessive amounts of ketone bodies in body tissues and fluids.

Lesion: Any pathological traumatic discontinuity of tissue or loss of function of a part.

Leukopenia: The numbers of leukocytes in the blood.

Leukemia: A progressive, malignant disease of the blood forming organs, marked by distorted proliferation and development of leukocytes and their precursors in the blood bone marrow.

Libido: The sexual drive, conscious, or unconscious.

Lymphocytosis: An excess of normal lymphocytes in blood or an effusion.

Malaise: Vagus feeling of discomfort.

Mastitis: Inflammation of the breast.

Menopause: Cessation of menstruation.

Metastasis: The process by which cancer spreads from the place at which it first arose as a primary tumor to distant locations in the body.

Metastasize: The spread from one part of the body to another. When cancer cells metastasize and cause secondary tumors, the cells in the metastatic tumor are like those in the original cancer.

Myalgia: Muscular pain.

Nausea: Tendency to vomit.

Necropsy: A postmortem examination or autopsy.

Necrosis: The death of living cells or tissues. Necrosis can be due, for example, to ischemia (lack of blood flow).

Neoplasia: The process of abnormal and uncontrolled growth of cells. The product of neoplasia is a neoplasm (a tumor).

Neoplasm: A tumor. An abnormal growth of tissue. The word neoplasm is not synonymous with cancer. A neoplasm may be benign or malignant.

Neuralgia: Paroxysmal pain extending along the course of one or more nerves.

Neuritis: Inflammation of nerves.

Nystagmus: Involuntary rapid movement of eyeball.

Oligospermia: decreased sperm count in serum.

Oliguria: decreased urine output in relation to fluid intake.

Ossification: Formation of or conversion into bone.

Ototoxic: Having a deleterious effect upon the eight nerve or on the organ of hearing and balance.

Palpitation: An awareness of the heart beat.

Palsy: Paralysis.

Pancytopenia: Abnormality of all cellular components of blood.

Parenteral: Administration by any way other than the mouth.

Paresthesia: Abnormal tingling sensation (pins and needles/ occurring spontaneously).

Pathology: The study of disease. Pathology has been defined as the branch of medicine which treats of the essential nature of disease.

Pancytopenia: A shortage of all types of blood cells, including red and white blood cells as well as platelets.

Pathognomonic: A sign or symptom that is so characteristic of a disease that it makes the diagnosis. For example, Koplik's spots (on the buccal mucosa opposite the 1st and 2nd upper molars) are pathognomonic of measles. The word "pathognomonic" (pronounced patho-no-monic) comes from the Greek "pathognomonikos' meaning skilled in judging diseases.

Peristalsis: A wave like movement that progressive along the intestines.

Pharyngitis: Inflammation of the part of the throat behind the soft palate.

Phobia: A physiological strong fear of a particular event or thing.

Prosthesis: Any artificial device that is attached to the body as an aid.

Purpura: A hemorrhagic area in the skin. The area of bleeding within the skin, by definition, is greater than 3 millimeters in diameter. The appearance of the purpura depends on age of the lesion. Early purpura is red and becomes darker, then purple, and brown-yellow as it fades. Purpura does not blanch when touched.

Raynaud's disease: A condition of unknown cause in which the arteries of the fingers are unduly reactive and enter spasm when the hands are cold.

Rhinitis: Inflammation of the mucous membrane of none.

Salpingitis: Inflammation of one or both of the fallopian tube caused by bacterial infection.

Side effects: Problems that occur when treatment goes beyond the desired effect. Or problems that occur in addition to the desired therapeutic effect. Example — A hemorrhage from the use of too much anticoagulant (such as heparin) is a side effect caused by treatment going beyond the desired effect.

Spasm: A brief, automatic jerking movement. A muscle spasm can be quite painful, with the muscle clenching tightly. A spasm of the coronary artery can cause angina. Spasms in various types of tissue may be caused by stress, medication, over-exercise, or other factors.

Spondylitis: Inflammation of the synovial joint of the backbone. Ankylosing spondylitis is a rheumatic disease involving the back bone and sometimes also causing arthritis in the shoulder and hip.

Syncope: Loss of consciousness due to temporary decrease in blood flow to brain.

Syndrome: A set of signs and symptoms that tend to occur together and which reflect the presence of a particular disease or an increased chance of developing a particular disease.

Tachycardia: Heart rate > normal rate.

Tachypnea: Resp. rate > normal rate.

Tenditis: Inflammation of a tendon.

Thromboembolism: The condition in which blood clot, formed at one point in the circulation, becomes detached and lodges at another point.

Trauma: A wound or injury, whether physical or psychic.

Tremor: A rhythmical alternating movement that may affect any part of the body.

Ulcer: A break in the skin or in the mucous membrane often accompanied by inflammation.

Vaginitis: Inflammation of vagina.

Vasodilatation: In diameter of blood vessel.

Vertigo: A disabling sensation in which the affected individual feels that either he himself or his surrounding in a state of constant movement.

Virilization: Induction of development of male secondary sex characters.

Vitiligo: A condition in which areas of skin lose their pigment and become white.

Western blot: A technique in molecular biology, used to separate and identify proteins.

APPENDIX 6

COMMONLY USED ABBREVIATIONS

AA	Amino acid
AB	Antibody
ABG	Arterial blood gases
AC	Adenylyl cyclase
ACE	Angiotensin-converting enzyme
ACh	Acetylcholine
ACHE	Acetylcholinesterase
ACTH	Adrenocorticotropic hormone
ADH	Antidiuretic hormone
ADS	Antidiphtheric serum
AF	Atrial fibrillation
AFB	Acid-fast bacilli
AGS	Antigasgangreno serum
AIP	Aldosterone-induced protein
ALL	Acute lymphoblastic leukaemia
AML	Acute myeloblastic leukemia
ANF	Antinuclear factor
APH	Antipartum hemorrhage
AR	Aortic regurgitation
ARC	AIDS-related complex
ARDS	Adult respiratory distress syndrome
ARF	Acute renal failure
ARS	Antirabies serum
AS	Aortic stenosis
ASD	Atrial septal defect
ASO	Antistreptolysin O
ATN	Acute tubular necrosis
ATS	Antitetanic serum
AZT	Zidovudine
BAL	British anti lewisite
BaMFT	Barium meal follow through
BBB	Blood-brain barrier
BBB	Bundle branch block
BCG	Bacillus Calmette Guerin
BHS	Benzene hexachloride
BMA	Bone marrow aspiration

BMT	Bone marrow transplant
BSA	Body surface area
BZD	Benzodiazepine
CA	Catecholamine
CAH	Chronic active hepatitis
CaM	Calmodulin
CAPD	Continuous ambulatory peritoneal dialysis
CAR	Conditioned avoidance response
CAT	Computerized axial tomography
CBF	Cerebral blood flow
CCB	Calcium channel blocker
CCU	Coronary care unit
CG	Chorionic gonadotropin
CHE	Cholinestrase
CHF	Congestive heart failure
CLD	Chronic liver disease
CLL	Chronic lymphoblastic leukemia
CMI	Cell mediated immunity
CML	Chronic myeloblastic leukemia
CMV	Cytomegalovirus
COPD	Chronic obstructive pulmonary disease
COX	Cyclooxygenase
CPS	Complex partial seizures
CPS	Complex partial seizures
CPZ	Chlorpromazine
CRF	Chronic renal failure
CRF	Corticotropin releasing factor
CT scan	Computerised tomographic scan
CTZ	Chemoreceptor trigger zone
CVA	Cerebrovascular accident
CVP	Central venous pressure
CWD	Cell wall deficient
CXR	Chest X-ray
DA	Dopamine
DAG	Diacyl glycerol
DAM	Diacetyl monoxime
DAMP	Diphenyl acetoxy-N-methyl piperidine methiodide
DAT	Dementia of Alzheimer type
DC shock	Direct-current shock
DEC	Diethylcarbamazine citrate

DHFA	Dihydrofolic acid
DIC	Disseminated intravascular coagulation
DIT	Diiodotyrosine
DM	Diabetes mellitus
DMPP	Dimethylphenylpiperazinium
DOSS	Dioctyl sodium sulfosuccinate
DOTS	Directly observed treatment strategy
DPT	Diphtheria-pertussis-tetanus (triple antigen)
E	Ethambutol
EBV	Epstein-Barr virus
ECG	Electrocardiogram
ECM	Ejection, systolic murmur
ECT	Electroconvulsive therapy
EDTA	Ethylene diamine tetra-acetic acid
EEG	Electrocardiogram
ELISA	Enzyme-linked immunosorbent assay
EMG	Electromyography
ERCP	Endoscopic retrograde cholangio pancreatography
ESR	Erythrocyte sedimentation rate
FFA	Free fatty acids
FFP	Fresh frozen plasma
FNAB	Fine-needle aspiration biopsy
FNAC	Fine-needle aspiration cytology
FSH	Follicle-stimulating hormone
GABA	Gamma-aminobutyric acid
G-CSF	Granulocyte colony stimulating factor
GFR	Glomerular filtration rate
GH	Growth hormone
GTCS	Generalized tonic-clonic seizure
GVH	Graft venous host disease
H or INH	Isonicotinic acid hydrazide (isoniazid)
HBV	Hepatitis B virus
HCV	Hepatitis C virus
HDL	High-density lipoprotein
HDV	Hepatitis delta virus
HIV	Human immunodeficiency virus
HLA	Human leucocyte antigen
HMW	High-molecular-weight
HOCM	Hypertrophic obstructive cardiomyopathy
HRT	Hormone replacement therapy

HSV	Herpes simplex virus
IBD	Inflammatory bowel disease
ICU	Intensive care unit
IE	Infectious endocarditis
IG	Immunoglobulin
IL	Interleukin
IP3	Inositol 1,4,5-triphosphate
IP4	Inositol tetratisphosphate
IPPR	Intermittent positive-pressure respiration
IPV	Inactivated polio vaccine
ITP	Idiopathic thrombocytopenic purpura
IU	International unit
IUCD	Intrauterine contraceptive device
IVP	Intravenous pyelogram
JVP	Jugular venous pulse
LA	Local anesthesia
LAH	Left anterior hemiblock
LBBB	Left bundle branch block
LDH	Lactate dehydrogenase
LDL	Low density lipoprotein
LMN	Lower motor neuron
LPH	Left posterior hemiblock
MAC	Minimal alveolar concentration
MAO	Monoamine oxidase
MBC	Minimal bactericidal concentration
MDI	Manic-depressive illness
MDM	Mid-diastolic murmur
MDT	Multidrug therapy
MHC	Major histocompatibility complex
MI	Myocardial infarction
MR	Mitral regurgitation
MRSA	Methicillin-resistant *Staphylococcus aureus*
MS	Mitral stenosis
MSH	Melanocyte-stimulating hormone
NLEP	National leprosy eradication programme
NMEP	National malaria eradication programme
NMR	Nuclear magnetic resonance
NSAID	Nonsteroidal anti-inflammatory drug
OC	Oral contraceptive
OGTT	Oral glucose tolerance test

OPV	Oral polio vaccine
OS	Opening snap
2-PAM	Pralidoxime
PABA	Para-aminobenzoic acid
PAF	Platelet-activating factor
PAH	Pulmonary artery hypertension
PAS	Para-aminosalicylic acid
PAT	Paroxysmal atrial tachycardia
PBI	Protein-bound iodine
PCP	Pulmonary capillary pressure
PCV	Packed cell volume
PDA	Patent ductus arteriosus
PEEP	Positive end-expiratory pressure
PG	Prostaglandin
PND	Paroxysmal nocturnal dyspnea
PNG	Penicillin G
PPD	Purified protein derivative
PPH	Postpartum hemorrhage
PPNG	Penicillinase producing N gonorrhoea
PSVT	Paroxysmal supraventricular tachycardia
PT	Prothrombin time
PUO	Pyrexia of undetermined origin
PV	Per vaginam
RA	Rheumatoid arthritis
RBBB	Right bundle-branch block
RBP	Retino-binding protein
RCU	Respiratory care unit
REM	Rapid eye movement (sleep)
RF	Rheumatoid factor
RHD	Rheumatic heart disease
RMP	Resting membrane potential
RVOT	Right ventricular outflow tract
S1	First heart sound
S2	Second heart sound
S3	Third heart sound
S4	Fourth heart sound
SABE	Subacute bacterial endocarditis
SC	Subcutaneous
SCC	Short-course chemotherapy

SIADH	Syndrome of inappropriate secretion of antidiuretic hormone
SLE	Systemic lupus erythematosus
SPS	Simple partial seizure
SRS-A	Slow-reacting substance of anaphylaxis
SVT	Supraventricular tachycardia
TAB	Typhoid, parathyroid A and B vaccine
THFA	Tetrahydrofolic acid
TIA	Transient ischemic attack
TOF	Tetralogy of Fallot
TR	Tricuspid regurgitation
TRH	Thyroid-releasing hormone
TS	Tricuspid stenosis
TSH	Thyroid-stimulating hormone
UDP	Uridine diphosphate
USG	Ultrasonography
UTI	Urinary tract infection
VBG	Venous blood gases
VC	Vital capacity
VDRL	Venereal disease research laboratory
VF	Ventricular fibrillation
VIP	Vasoactive intestine peptide
VLDL	Very low density lipoprotein
VSD	Ventricular septal defect
WHO	World health organization
WPW	Wolff-Parkinson-White syndrome
Z	Pyrazinamide

APPENDIX 7

WEIGHTS AND MEASUREMENTS OF ORGANS

1. Liver = 1500 gm = 1.8% of body wt.
2. Spleen = 150-200 gm = 0.16% of body wt.
3. Kidney = 130-160 gm.
4. Heart = 300 gm (in males), 250 gm (in females) = 0.45% of body wt.
5. Brain = 1400 gm 1.4% of body wt.
6. Right lung = 350-550 gm (Avg. 450 gm) 1% of body wt.
7. Left lung = 350-500 gm (Avg. 375 gm).
8. Spinal cord = 45 cm = 25 gm.
9. Pituitary gland = 0.5 gm.
10. Aortic valve (circumference) = 7.5 cm.
11. Pulmonary valve (circumference) = 8.5 cm.
12. Mitral valve (circumference) = 9.5 cm.
13. Tricuspid valve (circumference) = 10.5 cm.
14. Thyroid gland = 25 gm.
15. Thymus = 15-40 gm.
16. Trachea = 12 cm.
17. Pancrease = 100 gm = 0.1% of body wt.
18. Testis = 25 gm.
19. Prostate = 18 gm.
20. Uterus ⟨ Virgin = 30-40 gm.
    Parous = 100-120 gm.
21. Ovary = 8 gm.
22. Oesophagus = 25 cm.
23. Stomach = 25 cm= capacity is 1000 ml to 1500 ml.
24. Small intestine = 600 cm = 800 gm.
25. Large intestine = 150 cm = 600 gm.
26. Appendix = 8 cm.
27. Anal canal = 4 cm.
28. Urinary bladder = 25 cm = capacity is 250 ml.
29. Male urethra = 24 cm.
30. Female urethra = 4 cm.

31. Vagina $\Big\langle$ anterior wall = 8 cm

    posterior wall = 10 cm.
32. Placenta = 500 gm
33. Bones = 12% of body wt
34. Skeletal muscle = 38% of body wt
35. Pharynx = 12 cm

APPENDIX 8

DRUGS IN LACTATION

A. SAFE

1. Aspirin
2. Antacids
3. Beclofen
4. Cephalosporins
5. Codeine
6. Chromoglycate sodium
7. Diclofonac sodium
8. Digoxin
9. Erythromycin
10. Heparin
11. Ibuprofen
12. Insulins
13. Iron preparations
14. Lignocaine
15. Methyldopa
16. Paracetamol
17. Pyrazinamide
18. Salbutamol
19. Valproate sodium
20. Vitamins.

B. CONTRAINDICATED

1. Amiodarone
2. Amphetamines
3. Androgens
4. Anticancer drugs
5. Atropine
6. Chloramphenicol
7. Ciprofloxacin
8. Clindamycin
9. Cyclosporine
10. Ergotamine
11. Estrogens
12. Indomethacin

13. Ketoconazole
14. Lithium carbonate
15. Mefloquine
16. Tetracycline.

C. USE WITH SPECIAL PRECAUTIONS

1. Acyclovir
2. Aminoglycosides
3. Ampicillin/Amoxicillin
4. BZDs
5. Beta blockers
6. Chloroquine
7. Corticosteroids
8. Dapsone
9. Ethambutol
10. Furosemide
11. Isoniazid
12. Metochlopramide
13. Morphine
14. Nalidixic acid
15. Oral anticoagulants
16. Ranitidine
17. Rifampicin
18. Thyroxine
19. Sulfonylurea
20. Verapamil

APPENDIX 9

QUESTION PAPERS FOR PRACTICE

This question paper contains 2 printed pages.

7349   *Your Roll No..........*

II MBBS-2006 (Annual)

Paper I— PATHOLOGY – I

Time: 3 hours   *Maximum Marks: 40*

(Write your roll No. on the top immediately
On receipt of this question paper.)

Attempt all questions.
Use separate answer-books for parts I, II and III.
Attempt parts of a question in sequence.

PART-I

1. Differentiate between:
   (a) Necrosis and apoptosis
   (b) Primary and secondary amyloidosis
   (c) Iron deficiency anemia and Beta thalassemia trait
   (d) Antemortem thrombus and postmortem clot   8

2. Comment briefly on:
   (a) Role of human papilloma virus (HPV) in neoplasia
   (b) Spread of tumour
   (c) F VIII deficiency   6

PART-II

3. Write briefly on:
   (a) Lab diagnosis of cancer
   (b) Pathogenesis of septic shock   6

4. Write short notes on:
    (a) WHO classification of AML and their lab diagnosis
    (b) Laboratory diagnosis of multiple myeloma   6

PART-III

5. Write briefly on:
    (a) CSF findings in tubercular meningitis
    (b) Cytochemistry in acute leukemia
    (c) Prothrombin time
    (d) Primary complex   8

6. Write short notes on:
    (a) Indications and sites of bone marrow aspiration
    (b) Special stains for amyloid
    (c) Turner's syndrome.   6

This question paper contains 2 printed pages.

7350   *Your Roll No..........*

II MBBS-2006 (Annual)

Paper II— PATHOLOGY – II

Time: 3 hours   *Maximum Marks: 40*

(*Write your roll No. on the top immediately*
On receipt of this question paper.)

Attempt all questions.
Use separate answer-books for parts I, II and III.
Attempt parts of a question in sequence.

PART-I

1. Differentiate between:
   (a) Rheumatic and infective endocarditis
   (b) Benign and malignant nephrosclerosis
   (c) Tubercular and typhoid ulcer in intestine
   (d) Nephrotic and nephritic syndrome   8

2. Write briefly on:
   (a) Renal stones
   (b) Laboratory diagnosis of hepatitis B infection
   (c) Kimmel Steil-Wilson's disease   6

PART- II

3. Give brief account of:
   (a) Laboratory diagnosis of myocardial infarction
   (b) Sequelar of rheumatic heart disease   6

4. Write short notes on:
   (a) Etiopathogenesis of carcinoma colon
   (b) Pathogenesis of alcoholic liver disease   6

PART-III

5. Write gross and microscopic features of:
   (a) Bronchiectasis
   (b) Chronic pyelonephritis
   (c) Osteogenic sarcoma
   (d) Colloid goiter   8

6. Write briefly on:
   (a) Papillary carcinoma thyroid
   (b) Glioblastoma multiforme
   (c) Medullary carcinoma, breast   6

This question paper contains 2 printed pages.

7351   *Your Roll No..........*

II MBBS-2006 (Annual)

Paper III— MICROBIOLOGY

Time: 3 hours   *Maximum Marks: 40*

*(Write your roll No. on the top immediately
On receipt of this question paper.)*

*Attempt all questions.
Use separate answer-books for parts I, II and III.
Attempt parts of a question in sequence.*

PART-I

1. Define plasmids and describe transmission of plasmids among bacteria along with their application in drug resistance.   5

2. Write short notes on:
   (a) Bacterial capsule.   5
   (b) Antigen receptors on T-lymphocytes   5

PART – II

3. Describe laboratory diagnosis of secondary syphilis.   5

4. Discuss briefly:
   (a) Lab. diagnosis of meningitis caused by *Haemophilus influenzae.*
   5
   (b) Enterotoxigenic *Escherichia coli.*   5

PART – III

5. Presumptive coliform count.   5

6. Methods of toxin detection of *Corynebacterium dephtheriae*.

                                                                              5

This question paper contains 2 printed pages.

7352   *Your Roll No*..........

II MBBS-2006 (Annual)

Paper IV— MICROBIOLOGY

Time: 3 hours   *Maximum Marks: 40*

(Write your roll No. on the top immediately
On receipt of this question paper.)

Attempt all questions.
Use separate answer-books for parts I, II and III.
Attempt parts of a question in sequence.

PART – I

1. Describe briefly the morphology and life cycle of *Toxoplasma gondii.*   5

2. Write short notes on:
   (a) Cerebral malaria.   5
   (b) Life cycle of *Ascari lumbricoides*   5

PART – II

3. Enumerate causes of mycetoma and discuss the laboratory diagnosis of any of the fingal causes.   5

4. Write notes on:
   (a) Oral candidiasis.   5
   (b) Icosahedral virus symmetry.   5

PART – III

5. Enumerate arthropod-borne viruses commonly prevalent in India and describe laboratory diagnosis of any of them.   5

6. Strategies of HIV testing in India.   5

This question paper contains 2 printed pages.

7353   *Your Roll No..........*

II MBBS-2006 (Annual)

Paper V— PHARMACOLOGY – I

Time: 3 hours   *Maximum Marks: 40*

*(Write your roll No. on the top immediately
On receipt of this question paper.)*

*Attempt all questions.
Use separate answer-books for parts I, II and III.
Attempt parts of a question in sequence.*

PART – I

1. Explain why:
   (a) Half life of a drug varies for drugs undergoing zero order kinetics.
   (b) Digoxin is contraindicated in Wolf-Parkinson-White syndrome.
   (c) Atropine is preferred for refraction testing in children.
   (d) Pralidoxime is ineffective as antidote to carbamate poisoning.

   $2 \times 4 = 8$

2. Enumerate drugs for the treatment of congestive heart failure. Discuss the mechanism of action, therapeutic uses and adverse effects of Enalapril.   6

PART – II

3. Give rationale for the use of:
   (a) Carvidelol in heart failure
   (b) Diazepam in tetanus
   (c) Sodium bicarbonate in salicylate poisoning
   (d) Adenosine in supraventricular tachycardia. $2 \times 4 = 8$

4. Discuss the drug treatment of:
   (a) Status epilepticus
   (b) Migraine. $3 \times 2 = 6$

PART – III

5. Discuss the therapeutic status of:
   (a) Ephedrine in cough syrup
   (b) Tamsulosin in benign prostatic hypertrophy. $3 \times 2 = 6$

6. Write short notes on:
   (a) Polypharmacy
   (b) Drug tolerance
   (c) Pharmacovigilance $2 \times 3 = 6$

This question paper contains 2 printed pages.

7354   *Your Roll No.........*

II MBBS-2006 (Annual)

Paper VI— PHARMACOLOGY – II

Time: 3 hours   *Maximum Marks: 40*

(Write your roll No. on the top immediately
On receipt of this question paper.)

Attempt all questions.
Use separate answer-books for parts I, II and III.
Attempt parts of a question in sequence.

PART – I

1. Explain why:
   (a) Bisphosphonates are often prescribed to post-menopausal women.
   (b) Ketoconazole should not be used with cisapride.
   (c) Low molecular weight heparins are preferred over unfractionated heparin preparations.
   (d) Lispro insulin is used in infusion pump devices.

$$2 \times 4 = 8$$

2. Enumerate aminoglycoside antibiotics. Discuss their mechanism of action, anti-bacterial spectrum, therapeutics uses and side effects.   6

PART – II

3. Discuss rationale for the use of:
   (a) Finasteride in benign postatic hyperstrophy.
   (b) Progesterone with oestrogen in hormone replacement therapy.
   (c) Corticosteroids in ulcerative colitis.
   (d) Mifiprestone for termination of early pregnancy.

$$2 \times 4 = 8$$

4. Discuss the drug treatment of:
   (a) Peptic ulcer
   (b) Scabies   3 × 2 = 6

PART – III

5. Discuss therapeutic status of:
   (a) Folic acid in anaemia
   (b) 5 HT$_3$ antagonists in vomiting
   (c) Fluoroquinolones in tuberculosis.   3 × 2 = 6

6. Writ short notes on:
   (a) Irrational use of antimicrobial agents
   (b) Macrolide antibiotics
   (c) Selective oestrogen receptor modulators. 2 × 3 = 6

This question paper contains 2 printed pages.

7355   *Your Roll No..........*

II MBBS-2006 (Annual)

Paper VII— FORENSIC MEDICINE INCLUDING TOXICOLOGY

Time: 3 hours   *Maximum Marks: 40*

*(Write your roll No. on the top immediately
On receipt of this question paper.)*

*Attempt all questions.
Use separate answer-books for parts I, II and III.
Attempt parts of a question in sequence.*

PART – I

1. What are the findings, interpretation and medicolegal importance when it is stated that:
   (a) Death is due to traumatic asphyxia   2
   (b) Spalding sign is positive   2
   (c) A girl is of sixteen years of age   2
   (d) Burtonian's lines are present in a person   2

2. Write short notes on:
   (a) Cephalic index   2
   (b) Chelating agent   2
   (c) Inquest   2

PART – II

3. Classify neurotic poisons. Describe clinical features, management, postmortem findings and medicolegal significance in a case of Datura poisoning.   2

4. Differentiate between:
   (a) Suicidal and homicidal cut throat   2
   (b) Entry and exit of rifled firearm   2
   (c) Male and female mandible   2

PART – III

5. Define medical negligence. What are the various types of medical negligence along with various precautions a doctor should take to protect against such law suits?   7

6. Differentiate between:
   (a) Poisonous and non-poisonous snake   2
   (b) Antemortem and postmortem drowning   2
   (c) Dry heat burn and moist heat burn   2

This question paper contains 2 printed pages.

9255   *Your Roll No..........*

II MBBS-2007 (Annual)

Paper I— PATHOLOGY-I

Time: 3 hours   *Maximum Marks: 40*

*(Write your roll No. on the top immediately
On receipt of this question paper.)*

*Attempt all questions.
Use separate answer-books for parts I, II and III.
Attempt parts of a question in sequence.*

PART – I

1. Differentiate between:
   (a) Reversible and irreversible cell injury
   (b) Acute and chronic ITP
   (c) Dystrophic and metastatic calcification
   (d) Normoblast and megaloblast   8

2. Comment briefly on:
   (a) Lyon hypothesis
   (b) G6PD deficiency
   (c) Cell mediated hypersensitivity   6

PART – II

3. Write briefly on:
   (a) Paraneoplastic syndrome
   (b) Blood component therapy   6

4. Write short notes on:
   (a) Mode of transmission of HIV infection cut throat
   (b) Fate of thrombus   6

PART – III

5. Write briefly on:
   (a) Pathogenesis of septic shock
   (b) Pancytopenia
   (c) Mechanism of autoimmune disease
   (d) Down's syndrome   8

6. Write short notes on:
   (a) Philadelphia chromosome
   (b) Metaplasia
   (c) Osmotic fragility test   6

This question paper contains 2 printed pages.

9256   *Your Roll No..........*

II MBBS-2007 (Annual)

Paper II— PATHOLOGY-II

Time: 3 hours   *Maximum Marks: 40*

(Write your roll No. on the top immediately
On receipt of this question paper.)

Attempt all questions.
Use separate answer-books for parts I, II and III.
Attempt parts of a question in sequence.

PART – I

1. Differentiate between:
    (a) Tuberculous and amoebic ulcer
    (b) Dilated and hypertrophic cardiomyopathy
    (c) Lobar and bronchopneumonia
    (d) Type-I and Type-II Diabetes mellitus   8

2. Write briefly on:
    (a) Gallstones
    (b) Hydatidiform mole
    (c) Familial polyposis coli   6

PART – II

3. Write brief account of:
    (a) ARDS
    (b) Etiopathogenesis of emphysema   6

4. Write short notes on:
    (a) Barrett's oesophagus
    (b) Lung abscess   6

PART – III

5. Write gross and microscopic features of:
   (a) Carcinoma prostate
   (b) Seminoma
   (c) Meningioma
   (d) Renal cell carcinoma   8

6. Write briefly on:
   (a) Carcinoid syndrome
   (b) Causes of portal hypertension
   (c) Krukenberg's tumor.   6

This question paper contains 2 printed pages.

9257   *Your Roll No.*..........

II MBBS-2007 (Suppl.)

Paper III— MICROBIOLOGY

Time: 3 hours   *Maximum Marks: 40*

*(Write your roll No. on the top immediately
On receipt of this question paper.)*

*Attempt all questions.
Use separate answer-books for parts I, II and III.
Attempt parts of a question in sequence.*

PART – I

1. Describe briefly principle and functions of hot air oven.   5

2. Write short notes on:
   (a) IgM antibody   5
   (b) Adjuvants   5

PART – II

3. Classify mycobacteria. Write briefly about the laboratory diagnosis of pulmonary tuberculosis   5

4. Write short notes on:
   (a) TRIC agents   5
   (b) *Helicobacter pylori*   5

PART – III

5. Define biomedical waste. Discuss briefly its methods of disposal
   5

6. Describe briefly principle and uses of polymerase chain reaction (PCR)
   5

This question paper contains 2 printed pages.

9258   *Your Roll No..........*

II MBBS-2007 (Suppl.)

Paper IV— MICROBIOLOGY

Time: 3 hours   *Maximum Marks: 40*

*(Write your roll No. on the top immediately
On receipt of this question paper.)*

*Attempt all questions.
Use separate answer-books for parts I, II and III.
Attempt parts of a question in sequence.*

PART – I

1. Describe the life-cycle of malarial parasite in details.   5

2. Write short notes on:
    (a) Amoebic liver abscess   5
    (b) Casoni's test   5

PART – II

3. Name various genera of dermatophytes. Discuss the laboratory
    diagnosis of infections caused by dermatophytes   5

4. Write short notes on:
    (a) Rhinosporidiosis   5
    (b) Inclusion bodies   5

PART – III

5. Describe briefly various methods of viral cultivation   5

6. Discuss the laboratory markers associated with progession of HIV infection   5

This question paper contains 2 printed pages.

9259   *Your Roll No..........*

II MBBS-2007 (Annual)

Paper V— PHARMACOLOGY-I

Time: 3 hours   *Maximum Marks: 40*

(Write your roll No. on the top immediately
On receipt of this question paper.)

Attempt all questions.
Use separate answer-books for parts I, II and III.
Attempt parts of a question in sequence.

PART – I

1. Explain why:
   (a) Thiazide diuretics cause calcium retention while loop diuretics cause increase in calcium excretion
   (b) Ethanol is used in methanol poisoning
   (c) Plasma concentration of phenytoin rises disproportionately at higher doses
   (d) First dose of prazosin should preferably be administered at bed time $2 \times 4 = 8$

2. Classify antidepressant drugs. Write the mechanism of action, adverse effects and therapeutic uses of fluoxetine.   6

PART – II

3. Give rationale for the therapeutic use of the following:
   (a) Oximes in organophosphorus poisoning
   (b) Sumatriptan in migraine
   (c) Adenosine in the treatment of paroxysmal atrial tachycardia
   (d) Tizanidine in spastic disorders $2 \times 4 = 8$

4. Discuss the drug treatment of:
   (a) Status asthmaticus
   (b) Paracetamol poisoning $3 \times 2 = 6$

PART – III

5. Discuss the therapeutic status of:
   (a) ACE inhibitors in heart failure
   (b) Statins in dyslipidemia
   (c) Leukotriene antagonists in bronchial asthma $2 \times 3 = 6$

6. Write short notes on:
   (a) Fixed dose drug combinations
   (b) Drugs modulating cytochrome P_{450} enzymes
   (c) Drug-dependence $2 \times 3 = 6$

This question paper contains 2 printed pages.

9260   *Your Roll No..........*

II MBBS-2007 (Annual)

Paper VI— PHARMACOLOGY-II

Time: 3 hours   *Maximum Marks: 40*

(Write your roll No. on the top immediately
On receipt of this question paper.)

Attempt all questions.
Use separate answer-books for parts I, II and III.
Attempt parts of a question in sequence.

PART – I

1. Explain why:
   (a) Anaerobic microorganisms are resistant to aminoglycoside antibiotics
   (b) Heparin and Warfarin are started together in acute thrombo-embolic states
   (c) Thalidomide is used for lepra reaction
   (d) Dose of skeletal muscle relaxant should be lowered in patients receiving high doses of gentamicin $2 \times 4 = 8$

2. Classify drugs used in diabetes mellitus. Describe the pharmacology of oral hypoglycemic drugs   6

PART – II

3. Give rationale for the use of the following:
   (a) Hydroxy chloroquine in systemic lupus erythematosis
   (b) BAL in arsenic poisoning
   (c) Sildenafil in erectile dysfunction
   (d) Finasteride in prostatic disease $2 \times 4 = 8$

4. Discuss the drug treatment of:
   (a) HIV infection
   (b) MDR tuberculosis $2 \times 3 = 6$

PART – III

5. Discuss therapeutic status of:
   (a) Bisphosphonates in osteoporosis
   (b) Cyclosporine in renal transplants
   (c) Tamoxifen in breast cancer $2 \times 3 = 6$

6. Write short notes on:
   (a) Albendazole
   (b) Paclitaxel
   (c) Emergency contraceptives $2 \times 3 = 6$

This question paper contains 2 printed pages.

9261   *Your Roll No..........*

II MBBS-2007 (Annual)

Paper VII— FORENSIC MEDICINE INCLUDING TOXICOLOGY

Time: 3 hours   *Maximum Marks: 40*

*(Write your roll No. on the top immediately
On receipt of this question paper.)*

*Attempt all questions.
Use separate answer-books for parts I, II and III.
Attempt parts of a question in sequence.*

PART – I

1. What are the findings, interpretation and medicolegal importance when it is stated that :
   (a) Skull is having a ring fracture
   (b) Body is showing pugilistic attitude
   (c) Person is 12 years of age
   (d) Diatoms are present in bone marrow $2 \times 4 = 8$

2. Write short notes on:
   (a) Dying declaration
   (b) Whiplash injury
   (c) Privileged communication $2 \times 3 = 6$

PART – II

3. Classify irritant poisons. Describe clinical features, management, postmortem findings and medicolegal importance in a case of chronic mercury poisoning.   7

4. Differentiate between:
   (a) Dhatura and capsicum seeds
   (b) Burns and scalds
   (c) Antemortem and postmortem contusions $2 \times 3 = 6$

PART – III

5. Define rape. What will be findings in a 15 years old girl alleged to have been raped 12 hours ago? 7

6. Write short notes on:
   (a) Concussion
   (b) DNA fingerprinting
   (c) Impulse $2 \times 3 = 6$

APPENDIX IX

QUESTION PAPERS FOR PRACTICE

This question paper contains 2 printed pages.

1394

Your Roll No..........

II MBBS-2008 (Annual)

Paper I— PATHOLOGY – I

Time: 3 hours   *Maximum Marks: 40*

(Write your roll No. on the top immediately
On receipt of this question paper.)

Attempt all questions.
Use separate answer-books for parts I, II and III.
Attempt parts of a question in sequence.

PART-I

1. Differentiate between:
   (a) Healing by primary and secondary intention
   (b) Clonal deletion and Clonal anergy
   (c) Metaplasia and Dysplasia
   (d) CML and leukemoid reaction $2 \times 4 = 8$

2. Comment briefly on:
   (a) Laboratory diagnosis of diabetes mellitus
   (b) Down's Syndrome
   (c) Type III hypersensitivity reaction. $2 \times 3 = 6$

PART-II

3. Write briefly on:
   (a) Pathogenesis of fatty change liver
   (b) Component therapy $3 \times 2 = 6$

4. Write short notes on:
   (a) DIC
   (b) Laboratory diagnosis of tuberculous meningitis.   3 × 2 = 6

PART III

5. Write briefly on:
   (a) Opportunistic infections in AIDS
   (b) Laboratory diagnosis of beta-thalassemia
   (c) Radiation Injury
   (d) Factors affecting ESR   2 × 4 = 8

6. Write short notes on:
   (a) FAB classification of Acute Myeloid leukemia
   (b) Mechanics of Apoptosis
   (c) Etiopathogenesis of Shock   2 × 3 = 6

This question paper contains 2 printed pages.

1395   *Your Roll No..........*

II MBBS-2008 (Annual)

Paper II— PATHOLOGY – II

Time: 3 hours   *Maximum Marks: 40*

*(Write your roll No. on the top immediately
On receipt of this question paper.)*

*Attempt all questions.
Use separate answer-books for parts I, II and III.
Attempt parts of a question in sequence.*

PART I

1. Differentiate between:
   (a) Nephrotic and nephritic syndrome
   (b) Benign and Malignant Gastric ulcer
   (c) Rheumatic and bacterial endocarditis
   (d) Atheroma and Fatty Streak $2 \times 4 = 8$

2. Comment briefly on:
   (a) Prognostic factors in carcinoma breast
   (b) Clinical features and sequelae of Hepatitis B
   (c) Non-seminomatous germ cell tumours $2 \times 3 = 6$

PART-II

3. Write a brief account of:
   (a) Cushing syndrome
   (b) Osteogenic sarcoma $3 \times 2 = 6$

4. Write briefly on:
   (a) Hypersplenism and causes of splenomegaly
   (b) Cervical intraepithelial neoplasia $3 \times 2 = 6$

PART-III

5. Write briefly on:
   (a) Bronchogenic carcinoma
   (b) Krukenberg tumour
   (c) Barret esophagus
   (d) Wilms tumour $2 \times 4 = 8$

6. Write short notes on:
   (a) Complications of acute myocardia infarction
   (b) Etiopathogenesis and complications of gallstones
   (c) Neuroblastoma $2 \times 3 = 6$

This question paper contains 2 printed pages.

1396   *Your Roll No*..........

II MBBS-2008 (Annual)

Paper III— MICROBIOLOGY

Time: 3 hours   *Maximum Marks: 40*

(Write your roll No. on the top immediately
On receipt of this question paper.)

Attempt all questions.
Use separate answer-books for parts I, II and III.
Attempt parts of a question in sequence.

PART I

1. Describe the bacterial growth curve   5

2. Write short notes on:
   (a) Classical complement pathway   5
   (b) Monoclonal antibodies   5

PART-II

3. Describe the laboratory diagnosis of anaerobic infections. 5

4. Write short notes on:
   (i) The pathogenesis of acute rheumatic fever   5
   (ii) Laboratory diagnosis of primary syphilis   5

PART-III

5. Describe the principle of ELISA. Enumerate the various types with one example each.   5

6. What are nosocomial infections? What is the role of a microbiologist in their control?   5

This question paper contains 2 printed pages.

1397   *Your Roll No..........*

II MBBS-2008 (Annual)

Paper IV— MICROBIOLOGY

Time: 3 hours   *Maximum Marks: 40*

*(Write your roll No. on the top immediately
On receipt of this question paper.)*

*Attempt all questions.
Use separate answer-books for parts I, II and III.
Attempt parts of a question in sequence.*

PART I

1. Describe the life cycle and diagnosis of the agent causing hydatid disease.   5

2. Write short notes on:
   (a) The differences between plasmodium vivax and plasmodium falciparum on peripheral blood smear examination.   5
   (b) Larva Migrans   5

PART II

3. Discuss the opportunistic fungal infections in HIV/AIDS.

4. Write short notes on:
   (a) Cryptococcus neoformans   5
   (b) Direct demonstration of fungi in clinical samples.   5

PART III

5. Enumerate 3 viruses transmitted by mosquito. Discuss the laboratory diagnosis of any one of these.   5

6. Describe the principles and strategies for prevention and eradications of Poliomyelitis.   5

This question paper contains 2 printed pages.

1398   *Your Roll No...........*

II MBBS-2008 (Annual)

Paper V— PHARMACOLOGY – I

Time: 3 hours   *Maximum Marks: 40*

*(Write your roll No. on the top immediately
On receipt of this question paper.)*

*Attempt all questions.
Use separate answer-books for parts I, II and III.
Attempt parts of a question in sequence.*

PART I

1. Explain why?

    (a) Diazepam though a drug of choice for status epilepticus is not recommended for maintenance therapy of epilepsy.

    (b) Halothane is frequently combined with nitrous oxide for general anaesthesia.

    (c) Digoxin but not adrenaline is used in congestive heart failure.

    (d) Acetazolamide is not preferred as a diuretic agent. $2 \times 4 = 8$

2. Enumerate commonly used opioids. Write the mode of action, indications and contraindications for the use of morphine.   6

PART II

3. Give the rationale for the therapeutic use of the following:

    (a) Sidenafil in erectile dysfunction

    (b) Mannitol in cerebral oedema

    (c) Combining levodopa with carbidopa in parkinsonism

    (d) Dopamine in cardiogenic shock $2 \times 4 = 8$

4. Discuss the drug treatment of
   (a) Generalised tonic clonic seizures
   (b) Acute gout   3 × 2 = 6

PART-III

5. Discuss the therapeutic status of
   (a) Sodium chromoglycate in bronchial asthma
   (b) Clozapine in schizophrenia
   (c) Terlipressin in bleeding oesophageal varies   2 × 3 = 6

6. Write short notes on:
   (a) Therapeutic window
   (b) Midazolam
   (c) Bioavailability   2 × 3 = 6

This question paper contains 2 printed pages.

1399   *Your Roll No..........*

II MBBS-2008 (Annual)

Paper VI— PHARMACOLOGY – II

Time: 3 hours   *Maximum Marks: 40*

(Write your roll No. on the top immediately
On receipt of this question paper.)

Attempt all questions.
Use separate answer-books for parts I, II and III.
Attempt parts of a question in sequence.

PART I

1. Explain why?
    (a) Ondansetron is preferred over prochlor-perazine for the treatment of cancer chemotherapy induced emesis.
    (b) Ketoconazole is useful in treatment of Cushing's syndrome.
    (c) Dexrazoxane pretreatment is given with doxorubicin therapy.
    (d) Oxytocin and not ergometrine is used for augmenting the labour. $2 \times 4 = 8$

2. What is HAART? Write the mode of action, adverse effects and clinically important drug interactions of nevirapine   6

PART II

3. Give the rationale for the use of:
    (a) Propranolol in thyrotoxicosis
    (b) Filgrastim in cancer chemotherapy
    (c) Alendronate in osteoporosis
    (d) diloxanide furoate and metronidazole in amoebiasis
                                                          $2 \times 4 = 8$

4. Discuss the drug treatment of:
   (a) Chronic, recurrent urinary tract infection in females
   (b) Peptic Ulcer with H. pylori infection $2 \times 3 = 6$

PART III

5. Discuss the therapeutic status of:
   (a) Rosiglitazone in diabetes mellitus
   (b) Ivermectin in filariasis
   (c) Artemisinin in malaria $2 \times 3 = 6$

6. Write short notes on:
   (a) Plasma expanders
   (b) Post antibiotic effect
   (c) Emergency contraception $2 \times 3 = 6$

This question paper contains 2 printed pages.

1400   *Your Roll No..........*

II MBBS-2008 (Annual)

Paper VII— FORENSIC MEDICINE INCLUDING
TOXICOLOGY

Time: 3 hours   *Maximum Marks: 40*

*(Write your roll No. on the top immediately
On receipt of this question paper.)*

*Attempt all questions.
Use separate answer-books for parts I, II and III.
Attempt parts of a question in sequence.*

PART I

1. What are the findings, interpretations and medicolegal
    importance, when it is stated that:
    (a) Hydrostatic test is positive.
    (b) The death is due to traumatic asphyxia
    (c) Cadaveric spasm is present
    (d) The person is in lucid interval $2 \times 4 = 8$

2. Write short notes on:
    (a) Contributory negligence
    (b) True and Feigned mental illness
    (c) Counter coup injury $2 \times 3 = 6$

PART II

3. What are somniferous poisons? Describe the clinical features,
    management, postmortem findings and medicolegal significance
    in a case of acute morphine poisoning.   7

4. Differentiate between:
   (a) Entry and exit wounds of rifled firearm
   (b) Heat haematoma and extradural haematoma
   (c) Ligature marks of hanging and strangulation $2 \times 3 = 6$

PART III

5. Classify thermal injuries. Describe in detail the cause of death, postmortem findings in a case of carbon monoxide poisoning.

   7

6. Write short notes on:
   (a) Patterned injuries
   (b) Delusion
   (c) Hostile witness. $2 \times 3 = 6$